THE POWER

OF

MY-CHI

THE POWER

OF

MY-CHI

Tom Sullivan

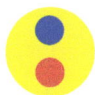

MY-CHI PUBLICATIONS

THE POWER OF MY-CHI
Text © Tom Sullivan 2015.
Photographs © Jack Malthouse 2015.
Published by My-Chi Publications, England.

ISBN 978-0-9933651-0-2

Tom Sullivan asserts his moral right to be identified as the author of this book.

ADVICE TO THE READER:
This book is not intended as a substitute for the medical advice of physicians. The reader should regularly consult a physician in matters relating to his/her health and particularly with respect to any symptoms that may require diagnosis or medical attention.

Before following any exercise in the program contained in this book, it is recommended that you consult your physician if you suffer from any health problems or special conditions or are in any doubt as to its suitability for your lifestyle.

CONTENTS

*This book is dedicated to the memory of my mother
Freda Mary Sullivan, the consummate story-teller.*

Teachers open the door; you enter by yourself.

Chinese proverb

ACKNOWLEDGEMENTS

When I finally decided to write the book *The Power of My-Chi*, I felt it was a path that I alone would need to walk. As I began this new adventure, good people appeared and walked beside me, assisting me unselfishly along the way. My deepest gratitude goes out to the following people for their encouragement, enthusiasm, professionalism, expertise and time given.

To my daughter Rebecca and son Gareth, both of whom have taken up the My-Chi lifestyle and exhibit their knowledge of the My-Chi exercises in the diagrams of this book.

To my good friend and student, 4th Dan Simon Brierley, for his consistent support and belief in My-Chi.

To Erzebet and Chris Carr, without whose help, professionalism and great knowledge of the writing, editing, and publishing world, this book may never have been able to reach the future practitioners of My-Chi. Gratitude! Gratitude!

To Jack Malthouse, whose faith in this project allowed it to flourish. Jack has proven himself to be highly technical and professional regarding the illustrations in this book. Jack has travelled along side me the whole way, my gratitude to him is endless.

I have met many good and beautiful people whilst writing and publishing this book.

Thank you all for being there.

Tom Sullivan

FOREWORD: A MESSAGE FROM TOM MY-CHI

Welcome to the harmony and balance of My-Chi.

My-Chi is for everyone who is looking for the first step of self-improvement. Young or old, abled or disabled, fit or unfit – Chi is within us all.

My-Chi has no boundaries, no limitations, no restrictions nor selective preference as to whom can benefit; we *all* can and will benefit from taking that first step.

Allow me to introduce you to your Chi and you will be truly amazed by the feeling of harmony and balance within your mind, body, and spirit, giving you an overall feeling of total wellbeing and the ability to achieve great things.

Once perfected the initial exercise will take no longer than several minutes. The results will undoubtedly speak for themselves.

There are no accessories required or expensive suits of clothing to purchase in order to practice My-Chi. Any loose-fitting attire will do perfectly.

The only thing needed is what we all have within ourselves – mind, body, and spirit – and the desire to take the first step to combine all three and thus become the best we can be, by way of My-Chi.

You must remember that when training My-Chi, you are in fact training and exercising *your* Chi.

Chi belongs to us all.

Tom My-Chi

Begin at the beginning...and go on till you come to the end: then stop.

Lewis Caroll, Alice in Wonderland

Introduction:
The Beginning

My name is Tom Sullivan, 5th Dan martial arts instructor. I am registered with N.A.K.M.A.S., the National Governing Body for British Martial Arts. My fundamental teachings originate from the style of Goju-Ryu, Japanese for "hard-soft style". It is one of the main traditional Okinawan styles of Karate. The major emphasis of Goju-Ryu is given to breathing correctly in all of the katas (choreographed patterns of movement), but particularly in the Sanchin kata, or the Three Battles kata, sometimes interpreted as the battle to unify the mind, body, and spirit.

I was raised in the City of Salford, now part of Greater Manchester in the North of England. I later moved to the North side of Manchester, to the town of Heywood, where I now live. Heywood is where my life's journey became an adventure, and an awakening as to the limitless possibilities that lay within myself to achieve.

At the age of twenty I was regularly attending a dermatology hospital on Quay Street in Manchester, as for the previous five years I had been suffering from the hereditary skin disease called psoriasis. I was classed as a chronic sufferer. Psoriasis restricted the quality of my life in many ways; for example my skin was extremely flaky and itchy and wherever I sat or stood there would be a deposit of skin left behind. I appeared to have extreme dandruff deposits on my collar and shoulders, and people would see the rash on my hands and face and ask if it was infectious. I was unable to do any form of sport because of this painful and embarrassing condition. I became a master of concealment in trying not to allow others to see that I had a major skin problem. At the time, psoriasis covered ninety percent of my body.

One day, my life was changed beyond all hope or expectation; I was offered the opportunity to reach for the stars and beyond, to be who and what I wished to be without the restrictions of psoriasis.

A skin specialist at the Quay Street Hospital on this momentous day informed me that a new treatment for psoriasis had been found. PUVA entailed taking Psoralen tablets that reacted to ultraviolet light. I was excited by the prospect of a possible cure for this cursed disease and decided without much consideration to accept the treatment. Within one week I could see the psoriasis disappearing from my body; within four weeks it had totally vanished and I must say that the ultraviolet light had given my skin a tan that looked rather attractive. Due to this newfound bodily freedom, I became much more positive in both mind and spirit and channelled my positive attitude into becoming physically fit and strong. At twenty-seven years of age I began training within the world of the martial arts.

I concentrated my mind, body, and spirit, deeply committing myself to the disciplines that were necessary in order for me to perfect the art that quickly became a passion and a way of life. My training paid dividends in a big way. I was looking good, feeling good, walking tall, I was full of confidence and my outlook was now positive, so much so that family and friends commented on the physical and spiritual change in me. This total transformation encouraged those around me to take up this type of training, and it was a pleasure to see their progression and their personal transformation as they worked alongside me. Within three years I had my own school with over a hundred students training regularly. I was a black belt 1st Dan and in the best physical, mental, and spiritual shape of my life.

It was never my intention to teach what I had learnt and found within the martial arts; it was for me something personal and self-fulfilling. When I look back, however, I feel fortunate to have had the privilege of teaching all of my students who were also searching for their *way* – a term I use quite often in this book and in my teachings which describes a student's path to reaching what they wish to achieve, or the road they choose to travel in order to progress and achieve their own personal goals.

For the following twenty-three years I trained and taught at an extremely high level within the martial arts; however, by the age of fifty my body had slowed down. I still felt good within myself, but I knew that to teach with enthusiasm and honesty at such a high level would, at that age, take a lot of commitment. I decided that it was time to hand over my school to my highest and most dedicated student.

Once I was no longer actively involved in the martial arts, I missed the feeling of inner strength that my training had generously given to me. My posture had dropped and I was no longer walking tall as I knew I ought to be doing.

This was also the age at which I retired from my position at the police force on the grounds of ill health. That along with certain events, including my private car being petrol-bombed, threats of many kinds towards my family and myself, the need for my home to be wired up with personal attack alarms, villains placing trackers on my private car, all played a major role in my descent into a deep depression, as well as causing me anxiety and stress.

On top of this, after I retired I noticed that I had acquired a few lumps on my body. I returned to the hospital where I had received the PUVA treatment, where the lumps were biopsied and proved to be cancerous. The cause was due to the amount of PUVA treatment I had received over the years. I now had to deal with skin cancer and psoriasis as the PUVA could no longer be part of my treatment. I was prescribed tablets to take as treatment for both complaints. For the following four to five years I went into a very dark place, one which I often hear others talk of who suffer from depression.

Throughout this dark period I did not train, nor did I look after myself very well. I drank a lot of alcohol and put on about two stone (twenty-eight pounds) in weight. My wife helped me carry the burden of my illness and my gratitude to her is so big that it would be impossible to measure, but I still found myself in a downward spiral.

At some point I must have hit the bottom of the pit. I could see where I had taken myself and I didn't like where I was – I wanted to live a better life than that. Positivity finally began to break through as I accepted that though I could not change the past nor the present, I *could* change the future.

A full five years of abstinence from regular training affects even the most natural of athletes and by fifty-five years of age, I could no longer step into the martial arts arena and expect to achieve anywhere near the excellent standard that I had enjoyed during the previous years. I knew that I was facing an uphill battle; I had been here before all those years ago. Now, twenty-eight years older, I wondered how – after always giving one hundred percent to my training and teaching – I could possibly achieve the standard that I expected of myself and be satisfied with the feeling of wellbeing that I wished to achieve.

I strongly believe that all of the events that happen in our lives are set before us: what is coming, is coming. We cannot stop what is coming, but we can learn to be strong enough to deal with a situation when it arrives. My situation had arrived and I set about developing a method of training that would improve my mental, physical, and spiritual wellbeing.

I looked back over my years in the martial arts, searching for the answers, looking for a way in which I could harness the power and feeling of wellbeing that I had felt whilst training for all of those years. I cannot truly say that I experienced a eureka! moment; I can however say that I dissected my knowledge of the martial arts, and from it pieced together a new revolutionary way of training based on breathing and slow movements that harnessed the energy source I knew lay within me and the whole of humankind. This energy source is known as *Chi* (pronounced as in *tea*).

Once perfected, this exercise became my first step to reclaiming the power of Chi I had felt all those years ago whilst training. My posture began to rapidly improve, I felt much stronger and more powerful, and I was once again the positive person family and friends had known me to be. I had been given a new lease on life.

This new form of exercise harnesses the power of Chi that is within us all. It takes only three minutes or less of coordinated breathing and light exercise and, once mastered, you too will see and feel a change within yourself.

Unwrap the gift of My-Chi, take it – it's yours for free. It has been there within you all along, waiting for you to unleash and enjoy the power of wellbeing.

One step at a time is good walking.
Chinese proverb

My-Chi on the Camino Santiago de Compostela

In January 2010, after writing the main essence of this book, I decided that I needed to exercise my own Chi and test my spiritual awareness. I was by now feeling good with the My-Chi exercises that I had developed, and was practicing them twice a day. I had lost the excess two stone that I had been carrying and was now down to thirteen and a half stone.

I was talking to a good friend of mine, a retired Army Major, and mentioned that I would like to take on a difficult challenge, perhaps walk the full length of Spain. He told me of the *Camino Santiago de Compostela*, a spiritual pilgrimage along the Frances (French) route that would begin for me in Roncesvalles at the foot of the Pyrenees in Spain and end in Santiago de Compostela, for a total of 780 kilometres (485 miles) along the western side of that beautiful country. This was the ideal opportunity for me to test the power of My-Chi and so I set about preparing for this walk of endurance across Northern Spain.

At 5:30 in the morning on May 1, 2010, in my sixtieth year on this earth, I arrived at Roncesvalles by taxi. The driver dropped me off outside a large building that looked rather spooky in the early hours of dawn. The taxi drove off into the direction of Pamplona, from where we had originally set off, leaving me alone in the darkness. It was very cold and, surprisingly, there was snow on the ground. It was deathly quiet and I wondered what to do next.

I then noticed to the left of the building a large oak door. I stood outside and listened at the door but there was not a sound from within. I turned the handle opened the door and stepped inside, where I saw, by the low lights, rows of double-decked bunk beds all full with what I presumed to be sleeping pilgrims.

To my left there were about five tables lined up end to end. A man seated behind the centre table beckoned me over, and explained that the pilgrims would shortly be rousing and preparing for the day's walk. He issued me with my *Credencial*, the official document of the pilgrim, in exchange for three euros, and invited me to go down into the basement where I could get a drink from the vending machine. Other pilgrims shortly began coming down for breakfast and before long there was a buzz of excitement as they prepared for the walk ahead.

When I left the building it was clear daylight and some pilgrims were already making their way along the track. I had now been awake for over twenty hours. I performed the My-Chi exercises at the beginning of the trail and despite the lack of sleep, I felt good and energised on this cold but sunny morning. The exercises had given me a much needed boost.

At 7:00a.m. I set off walking. I had a backpack that weighed thirteen kilograms containing what I believed were my essentials for a thirty-five day walk: sleeping bag, sandals, first aid kit, toiletries, head torch, three tee-shirts, three pairs of socks, three pairs of boxer shorts, three pair of trousers, one litre of water, an apple, a pear, a towel, pillow case, camera, documents, maps, sun cream, sun glasses, and other small items I might need along the way.

For those who speak many languages, this is the place to be. The Camino is a universal pilgrimage known to people from all over the world: Canadians, Japanese, South Koreans, Americans, French, Germans, Spanish of course, but no British…except for me. These others each had their own reasons for their pilgrimage – some spiritual, some trying to find their way in life or looking for answers, others just enjoying the challenge of the walk itself. Before long I realised that most of them were on the Camino for perhaps a week or two at the most – they were doing it over a period of years. I was one of only the few that was in it to the end in one full stretch.

Each day the weather was extremely hot and by the mid-afternoons it was up to around ninety degrees fahrenheit out there on the Camino. Each night I stopped and slept in *albergues*, hostels reserved especially for pilgrims. Sometimes there were thirty of us to a room, other nights only four. At the *hostales* (hotels) you have to pay

　　　　　　　　　　　　　　THE POWER OF MY-CHI

extra, however it was worth it just to have a private bathroom and not to have to listen to people snoring as you had a room to yourself.

Every day of the Camino I did my exercises in the mornings, before setting off, and in the evenings, just before bed. There were times that I felt totally exhausted whilst walking and I would stop take off my pack and do My-Chi exercises for about three minutes, after which I would drink some water pick up my pack and carry on totally rejuvenated.

I was averaging twenty-five kilometres (approximately sixteen miles) each day; however, blisters had developed early in my walk and by the seventh day I needed to treat them. Though my feet were sore, I continued training with My-Chi, and each morning after training I set off with a positive attitude. After two weeks and approximately three hundred and fifty kilometres my feet began to mend. I had lost about a stone in weight by this time and my pace had improved considerably.

My fellow pilgrims were quite curious about My-Chi, some noticing the change in my energy levels that were enabling me to maintain a positive attitude on what was a challenging journey. Often pilgrims asked me if I would teach them the moves. I began the lessons with the breathing and then, following my example, they joined me in the movements. Afterwards, they told me how much they enjoyed the feeling it gave them. I certainly enjoyed teaching them.

On June 1st I arrived in Santiago de Compostela, thirty-two days after setting off from Roncesvalles. I had walked on average of just under twenty-five kilometres a day. I was two stone lighter in weight, I was rather dishevelled, and when I look now at the photos that were taken on that journey, I also appeared painfully thin though at the time I hadn't noticed.

I must say that I felt a sense of spirituality upon my arrival. The story goes that Saint James, Jesus's disciple, is interred in the cathedral at Santiago de Compostela. There is a crypt below the main altar at the rear; visitors walk through a little passageway into a small area where they can kneel at the opening of the crypt, where Saint James's cask is visible behind an iron gate. Many pilgrims take their turn to kneel and sometimes pray or talk to the saint.

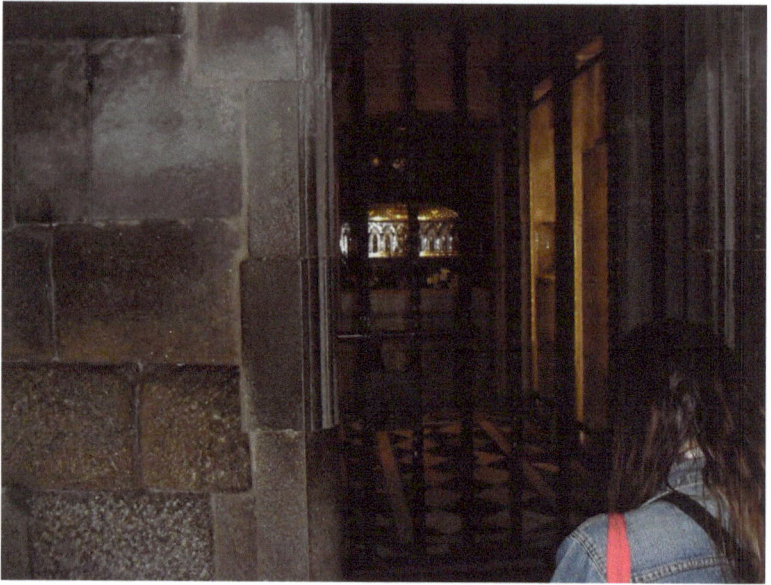

A YOUNG LADY PRAYS AT THE CRYPT

I knelt and asked the saint for a few things myself, favours for others that I knew were suffering, and also for others who were strong believers of the faith that had asked me to mention theirs or their loved ones' problems. Whether you believe or do not believe, it doesn't appear to matter in the Cathedral of Santiago; there is a strong sense of hope and joy for all who enter.

At the end of this journey I knew I had developed My-Chi into a powerful and strong exercise. I was totally focused and the feeling of wellbeing was now firmly a part of my way of life. I would not allow a day to go by without the feel good factor of My-Chi entering my whole being. I began walking the occasional sixteen kilometre (ten miles) walk two or three times a week around the local area where I lived. This helped me remain focused; walking had now become a part of my life that I enjoyed.

As time went by I felt the need to test once again the power and positivity that My-Chi had given me. I decided that I would walk the Camino Santiago de Compostela again, this time by a greater and more difficult route and over a longer period of time.

On May 1st 2012 I set off walking the northern route of the Camino Santiago, the *Camino Norte*, along the western coastline of Spain.

The Camino Norte starts at the foot of the Pyrenees Mountains in Irun and travels 820 kilometres to Santiago de Compostela. The route takes you along the western coastline of Spain, initially walking through Basque Country, San Sebastian up until Bilbao and then onto Santander. The terrain is rugged and steep which makes it a difficult walk to begin with.

The Northern route is not as spiritual as the Frances; it is seen more of taking the challenge as opposed to taking the pilgrimage. The Frances is the original route of the pilgrim and the Norte was later developed when the Moors invaded Spain, pushing the prospective pilgrims to the outer northern edges of Spain in order to avoid conflict.

The Camino Norte took me thirty-two days to complete in total. My-Chi worked its magic once again; however, on this occasion everything was balanced – mind, body and spirit – and when I arrived in Santiago I felt fit enough to walk back to Irun. I knew from that moment on that with My-Chi in my life I would constantly be looking for further challenges, and on May 1st, 2013, I decided to walk the hardest Camino, the *Camino del Sureste*, from its beginning in Alicante, Spain, as far as to where it meets the French route, the Camino Frances, in Astorga – nine hundred kilometres in total.

I made a slight alteration at the beginning of this Camino, starting in San Pedro on the Costa Blanca, instead of Alicante. I was the first person ever to take this route as I cut across to Orihuela, Abanilla, Pinoso, and then onto Yecla on the main Alicante Sureste route. I mention this Camino as one of many strange things happened to me on this thirty-six day walk. After about twenty-two days I hadn't met many other pilgrims and certainly had not spoken English, my native tongue, to any other native English speaking person.

It is a strange phenomenon to experience the lack of communication with a fellow native speaking person, and while there are those of other nationalities that speak very good English on these Caminos, it somehow does not fill that void that develops within oneself after a while. Loneliness and endurance combined can have a profound effect on a person; whilst My-Chi was giving me the energy and the determination I needed to walk this Camino, my mind was emptying itself of material thoughts and the familiar indoctrinations that I knew to be comforting and true.

Whilst walking along a path of pebbles, some large, some small, all different in size and colour, I noticed one particular pebble that stood out among the thousands that lay there. I picked up the pebble and held it between my index finger and my thumb. Its texture felt good to the touch. I carried on walking, rubbing the pebble without thought – almost in a Zen-like way. I decided that the pebble would accompany me to Astorga and that I would then take it home as a memento of my walk on the Camino.

Eight days later I noticed by the wayside a small pile of pebbles, obviously built by pilgrims passing through. On the top was a large pebble the size of a tennis ball. I felt the urge to leave the pebble I had found on top of the pile. To my amazement, there was a groove in the large pebble into which my pebble fit perfectly, as though mine was the missing piece.

I stood for a while looking at this pile of pebbles that pilgrims had left, perhaps in memory of a loved one, or as a prayer to help a loved one overcome an illness, or perhaps for themselves as a spiritual meaning. My pebble lay there because it belonged there with all those other pebbles that were placed there by pilgrims with belief and hope.

After thirty-six days and nine hundred kilometres I arrived in Astorga and stayed in the Pension Garcia where I had been before when on the Camino Frances. I was there for two days, gathering my thoughts and writing down my feelings towards this Camino and how it may have affected me. My conclusion was that of great satisfaction after walking the hardest walk of my life.

My-Chi was with me all the way. I developed self-confidence, an attitude of power and energy, and a feeling of gratitude for what was around me: the fresh air, the warm sunshine, and the kind friendly people that had helped me along the way with their accurate directions. I had slept in churches, sports halls, colleges, and at one time with a family who generously gave me shelter in their home.

Doing My-Chi exercises daily gave me a feeling of total wellbeing. I was positive and others had picked up on that positivity, seeing a person that was self-assured and in command of his own fate.

My-Chi is now my way and my life, and my wish now is to pass this way of My-Chi on to others, for them to have the opportunity to experience the power and well-being of My-Chi, to exercise the combination of mind, body and spirit. We all have it and owe it to ourselves to embrace that which lays within us – My-Chi.

Conflict cannot survive without your participation.
Wayne Dyer

BUILDERS AND DESTROYERS

Throughout my time as a self-defence instructor, I have seen thousands of students come and go from my club. I could initially separate the students into two categories: builders of obstacles, and destroyers of obstacles. The builder of obstacles would talk about why he or she couldn't manage one hundred push-ups in the class because of a sore arm, whilst the destroyer of obstacles would talk about how good the session was as he or she was pushed to their limits. This type of attitude can also be seen in the everyday life of the general public.

I wish to share with you my thoughts on builders of obstacles and destroyers of obstacles, as I truly believe that to place an obstacle in front of yourself is to deny yourself the whole essence of life and its mysteries.

There are many obstacles in our lives that appear to prevent us from achieving our goals, or perhaps deny us the opportunities that are offered to or acquired by others. Let's consider three types of obstacles:

- Obstacles that are set before us by life itself; they challenge us with daily problems that we must address.
- Obstacles that test us and hopefully develop our resolve and character.
- Obstacles that are self-imposed. These obstacles give us an excuse not to progress, not to achieve what others have achieved or aspire to achieve.

Now let's look at the destroyers and the builders of obstacles.

The Destroyer

Destroyers have no need to consider the third type of obstacle (self-imposed) as they focus on destroying the first type, the obstacles with which life itself confronts them. They enjoy life's challenges and meet them head on; they become skilled in preventing these obstacles from getting in the way of their progress. The second type of obstacle could be a physical impairment, a lack of education, or a poor background that excludes them from certain prospects and so on. We all know people who have destroyed this type of obstacle in all walks of life.

The destroyer achieves success because obstacles are not allowed to materialize and upset the equilibrium of his or her life's progress and ambitions.

The Builder

The builder of obstacles deals with life's obstacles by avoiding them. These obstacles inevitably build up into a series of barriers that restrict access to opportunity. They become bigger and more plentiful, making life appear restrictive and oppressive, causing great stress and anxiety for the builder.

The second type of obstacle for the builder would be the exact same as that of the destroyer and yet provoke the exact opposite reaction. The builder will have an excuse ready to use and walk away, leaving the obstacle there, never to be approached again. The builder also has the third type of obstacles to deal with – the self-imposed obstacles, which because of the speed and ease with which they can be erected are plentiful in the life of the builder.

For example:

I would join the gym if I had the time and money.

I would have tended the garden had it not rained all summer.

I didn't get the promotion at work – I appear to miss out every time to a junior or less qualified person.

Excuses build more obstacles. They also upset the balance in your life – building obstacles has a negative impact on your outlook and prospects, and excuses will deny you the opportunity to progress. Success and achievement will always be distant aspirations for the builder.

Destroy your obstacles now and your life will become easier and much more rewarding as you reach your goals. You will feel positive in all that you do, which will increase your self-confidence, giving you the feeling of self-control over your own life and ambitions.

Be a
Destroyer of obstacles as in DOOer.
And not a
Builder of obstacles as in a BOOer.

My-Chi is the first step along the way of becoming a DOOer

Help people become more motivated by guiding them
to the source of their own power.

Paul G Thomas

WALK TALL

There are many problems in our lives that seem to be outside of our control. They appear insurmountable, unsolvable, and at times take over any possible feeling of well-being. Outside influences could be bullies who make our lives a living hell, be it in the workplace, in our social lives, or even within our own close family. Some nasty-minded people, for no apparent reason, just may not like us. They might become vindictive towards us, making us feel small, hopeless or helpless, leaving us no way of escaping their negative intentions.

We have an entitlement to feel positive and happy with our lives, and it is up to us to make it so.

Consider this – you may not be able to control those outside influences, but you can one hundred percent control the influences that you have allowed to be imposed upon yourself. You can do this by learning to walk tall.

How do I walk tall? How can I alter my life for the better and change my present situation, making myself feel stronger, more assertive, and more confident around others?

The first step to walking tall is to believe in one's self. Take a good, honest look at who and what you are, have a full self-appraisal and accept that you have weaknesses and faults. Recognize them because others will have seen and recognized them and will possibly use them against you. Stress, depression, anxiety, lack of self-confidence can make a person a possible target for those that are looking for a victim. Now is the time to be rid of those weaknesses and faults. Write them down candidly, analyse them, dissect them, and by doing so release oneself from the shackles. From that point you must begin to develop your strengths, which of course are much easier for you to accept than are the criticisms of others regarding your weaknesses.

Develop your strengths with My-Chi and after a short period of time you will be rid of your weaknesses. The strength of mind, body, and spirit will take you where you wish to go. It will reveal a person of inner power and confidence, it will assist in good decision-making, and it may even rid you of those who are having a negative influence on your life.

If you have been lazy by nature, become industrious. If you have been a shy person, then become confident. Take the initiative and see how your life changes for the better. Walking tall will take time. Do it gradually and incorporate strengths along the way. Weaknesses, on the other hand, must go immediately. Do not blame others for your shortcomings. Accept the responsibility for and the consequences of your actions – empower your decisions, and confidently learn from your experiences.

If you win the race, you accept the adulation poured upon you for your personal success. If you lose the race, do not blame the weather, your trainers, or create any other excuse. Acknowledge that you gave it your best effort. Be true to yourself and accept that you gave it your all, and that sometimes your all isn't enough.

Walking tall, as you have probably gathered at this stage, is not about the height of the person. It concerns confidence, self-control, and a self-assured attitude. A person that walks tall can make responsible decisions, will exhibit true character, good manners, and consideration for others, and will ultimately be a person of inner strength.

A soon as you begin to train My-Chi you will understand, after feeling the power within yourself, what I mean by walking tall. You will experience confidence, positivity, and self-control. You will no longer fear challenges, you will embrace them.

In order to overcome your fears, you must confront them.

Nancy Musick

About My-Chi

Chi (氣) is a Chinese word used to describe the natural energy of the universe. One of the main concepts of Chi is that of harmony, whether in the universe or in the body. Disharmony causes imbalance and chaos, leaving a need for equilibrium. Chi can restore that balance.

For the practitioner of My-Chi, the word Chi means energy cultivation. My-Chi is an exercise formulated to combine mind, body, and spirit in order to create balance or equilibrium within yourself. This balance will give you a feeling of power and wellbeing, delivered by practicing a system of training techniques that develop physical and mental health by coordinating breathing exercises with physical movements and focus. Initially it takes no more than three minutes to complete the training program.

The Mind

Whereas the body can physically move things, and through the body the spirit can enhance that power, the mind is the most powerful when using all three in unison.

The healthy mind can achieve many things; however, the unhealthy mind is also powerful and could be counterproductive to the body and spirit, thus affecting our wellbeing. We must train the mind to become healthy by regularly organizing and exercising the body and spirit, thereby creating harmony and equilibrium within our whole being.

The first step in training the mind is through the exercise of My-Chi techniques, which teach the mind to exercise the body and spirit together in harmony. This fosters the natural balance of all three components which will provide the practitioner of My-Chi with a strong and positive outlook toward life.

THE BODY

The body is the vessel in which we carry our mind and spirit. The mind controls and protects the body, ensuring that it does not exceed its own capabilities; however, there are times when the body must bypass the mind, and in such cases the spirit will supersede any of the mind's instructions. In these cases, the body will exercise its unrestricted spiritual freedom, thus allowing it to utilize its full potential.

This untrained phenomenal burst of spiritual energy, or Chi, occurs only in highly exceptional circumstances. Many people have heard the story of the elderly lady lifting the car off her husband's chest with a supernatural power, thus saving his life. Chi is the essence of that power. My-Chi will provide you with the ability to harness and manifest this power, without overriding the mind, giving complete control of that power and energy as a result of mind, body, and spirit working as one.

It is of major importance to look after your body through good exercise, diet, and lifestyle; it is equally important to look after the inner organs of the body, to rid the body of bad toxins and to purify the blood that travels through every living structure of your body.

Studies have shown that the main killing diseases of our bodies in western countries (heart attack, stroke, cancer, and thrombosis) are connected with the way of life in our advanced urban societies, and that none of these diseases are as common among elderly people in underdeveloped countries. Thousands of research studies have shown that bad diet, smoking, lack of exercise, and temperament all have an influence on our overall physical health.

My-Chi will take away the stresses of life through accurate breathing techniques controlled by many various physical movements. The physical part of My-Chi enables you to control your breathing with greater accuracy, giving you the ability to concentrate the breathing at whatever level you wish without over-exerting yourself. It is essential that the breathing and the movements are coordinated and timed to perfection in order to acquire the best results.

You must first of all learn the My-Chi training position. When you feel quite proficient, you must then learn the breathing techniques, and then finally you must learn the body movements. When you feel ready to combine all three techniques, only then will you be prepared and able to begin the true exercise of My-Chi.

There is no great rush to combine the three techniques; practice well one technique and only when you feel confident with it should you then move on to the next technique and so on. I cannot stress often enough the importance of accuracy at the beginning, as faults will later be difficult to erase when they become habits. Achieving the right techniques from the outset will ensure that all basics are correct and will guarantee that all subsequent exercises are being done on a firm and true foundation.

THE SPIRIT

The spirit can be defined in many ways. For instance, there is the spirit of the individual who has shown exceptional courage in a life-threatening or highly dangerous situation. There is also the spirit of the person who overcomes adversity because of their tenacity. The spirit of My-Chi is a process of cultivating a controlled power and energy that is used to improve our lives and wellbeing. This spirit, when used in unison with the mind and body, gives the practitioner of My-Chi controlled and effective power which can be used as and when required.

When you become a member of the My-Chi family and you have learnt well the Cross, Wall, and Orb and feel the pure essence of My-Chi, you will find that it is an awakening to a new world, not only externally but also within yourself. You will see life from a totally different perspective – you will walk taller, think bigger, take on new challenges, and test your newfound inner strength, not just physically but also mentally and spiritually.

If you are at the peak of fitness and in very good health, My-Chi will give you the edge you've been looking for. Power, balance, speed, endurance – whatever it is, My-Chi will provide it for you. My-Chi will also help you prior to exams, interviews, and many other nerve-wracking encounters you may face throughout your lifetime. Once you become a student of My-Chi, it will take you approximately three minutes to acquire the inner strength you need on those occasions.

My-Chi is enjoying something that exists inside all of us and is all around us, no matter where we are, no matter who we are. There are no boundaries, so take that which belongs to you – Your-Chi.

We are spirits clad in veils.
Christopher Cranch

KNOW THE BODY
THAT YOU ARE IN

It is important that prior to beginning these exercises you become aware of your own body and its capabilities. Although the exercises are reasonably basic in the physical sense, I would ask that you follow the simple instructions below, for the sake of knowing for certain that you are fully bodily aware of any possible physical problems that may be revealed that restrict the initial exercises of My-Chi.

All of the following exercises are to be carried out gently and in a controlled fashion. During each exercise, pay attention to any feelings of restriction or discomfort.

Fingers: clasp and unclasp slowly five times.

Wrists: rotate the hands clockwise and anticlockwise five times.

Arms: rotate at full stretch at the side of the body in a circular fashion backwards and forwards slowly, left arm five times and then right arm five times.

THE FIRST STEP IS THE MOST DIFFICULT
OF ANY JOURNEY

POSTURE AND BREATHING

First of all, you must take up the correct posture. Place your feet shoulder-width apart with your knees slightly bent, shoulders back, chin up, and eyes focused straight ahead.

In order to acquire the full benefit of your exercise, it is important that you feel relaxed and comfortable in your new training posture. Practice stepping in and out of your training posture until you can adopt the position naturally.

Now that you have found your training posture and feel comfortable in your stance, breathe in deeply through the nostrils, fill your lungs with freshly oxygenated air, hold for approximately two seconds, and then force the air out of your lungs through a wide-open mouth using your diaphragm (the main muscle of respiration) to exert the pressure. Check your training posture and if your stance is correct, repeat the breathing exercise, this time with two repetitions: breathe in through the nostrils, hold the air in your lungs for approximately two seconds, and then exhale. Use the diaphragm to force the air out of your lungs as before, and then repeat the exercise one more time.

If you are feeling light-headed, wait until you feel confident enough to continue and only then proceed with the second exercise.

Relax and step out of your training posture and shake off. By this I mean move your hands and legs slightly, relaxing the muscles and breathing normally. When you are ready, step back into your training posture, correct your stance and check that you have not forgotten the main rules of the posture: feet shoulder-width apart, knees slightly bent, shoulders back, chin up, and eyes focused straight ahead.

Breathe in, hold for approximately two seconds and breathe out. Repeat two more times. Check your training posture. If it remains in the same correct position, then relax. If you have lapsed, then correct your posture and repeat the exercise until you are satisfied that the breathing is not affecting your stance.

It is important at this very crucial stage of your training in My-Chi that you rectify any faults in your posture and breathing.

There may be those who try too hard in one area, thus causing weakness in another. You must practice your training posture individually and you must practice your breathing individually, then combine the two and ensure they are working in total harmony. Only when you have mastered both will you feel the benefit of wellbeing that is beginning to run through your body, giving you the true feeling of Your-Chi.

Your-Chi

Once you have the training posture coordinated with the breathing, it is time to introduce body coordination. These movements are the key to summoning your Chi.

You must not do the body movements at the cost of the training posture or breathing exercises as this would be a backwards step and would affect your overall form.

Step into your training position. Check your stance (knees, shoulders, chin) and focus straight ahead. Do five breathing exercises, in through the nostrils, hold in the lungs for approximately two seconds, exhale through a wide open mouth, pushing with the diaphragm and then repeat the exercise a further four times.

Now stand in your training position with your closed hands pulled back and placed at the side of your ribs [see diagrams 1-2]. Take a deep breath through the nostrils, hold in the lungs for approximately two seconds and, immediately before exhaling, turn your hands into an open push position and push forward at shoulder height, forcing out the air through your open mouth as your arms become fully extended.

Slowly pull your arms back, closing your hands and breathing in through the nostrils. Return the closed hands to the side of your ribs. Hold your breath for approximately two seconds and repeat the exercise, turning your hands into an open push position, pushing forward at shoulder height, forcing the air out through the open mouth as the arms become fully extended.

Practice this well: rotate the hands from closed to open immediately prior to exhaling through the mouth, then extend the arms fully. Your exhalation must end at the exact moment your arms become fully outstretched. As you breathe in, retract your arms. Your lungs must be full at the exact moment your closed hands return to the side of your ribs.

Practice all that you have learnt so far, coordinating training posture, breathing, and movement. If you look through the diagrams in this book you will see that the Cross, Wall, and Orb exercises all begin after the initial intake of breath with the closed hands at the side of the ribs. It is important that you spend time now correcting any mistakes or bad habits before moving on to the full exercise of My-Chi.

When you have mastered the art of exercising My-Chi through what will become a natural habit for your mind, body, and spirit, you will then have the ability to concentrate that power and use it in many ways to improve and enhance your life.

One does what one is; one becomes what one does.
Robert Von Musil

Welcome to the World of My-Chi

The Cross

The Cross is the first set of techniques in which you will train. It consists of basic movements and will allow you to develop your Chi within a short period of time. As you progress eventually onto the Orb you will learn how to control and concentrate your Chi upon whatever object or part of your body you wish.

Some of the immediate effects of training the Cross are as follows:

Improved posture
Controlled breathing
Upper body toning
Stress relief
Feel more positive
Physical/mental strength
More energized
More confident
Improved general fitness

If you practice regularly, you will feel the energy of My-Chi flow through you; the balance of mind, body, and spirit will give you a wealth beyond any worldly fortune.

Forward Point

Adopt the training posture. Keep your eyes focused straight ahead throughout the exercise.

With your hands open and arms fully stretched at waist height as shown in diagram 1, pull your arms back to the closed-hand position at the side of the ribs and whilst doing so take in a deep breath through the nostrils.

Fill your lungs and hold for approximately two seconds, as shown in diagram 2.

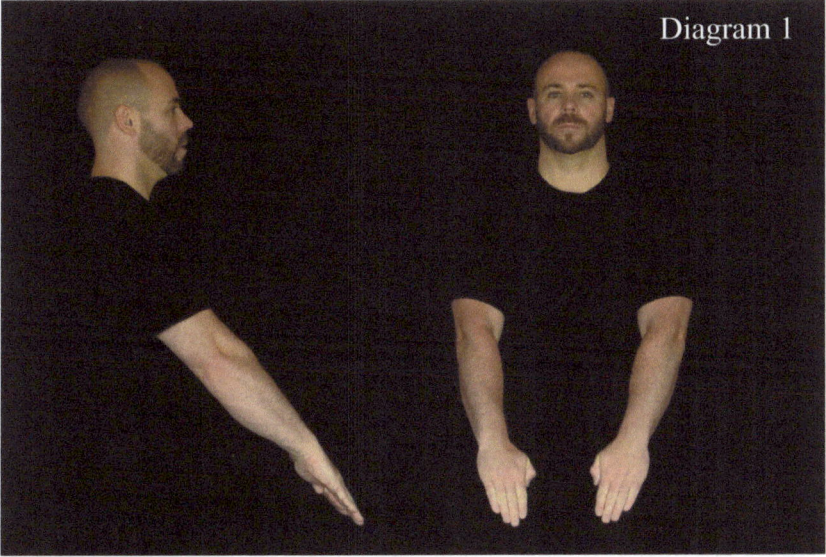

Diagram 1

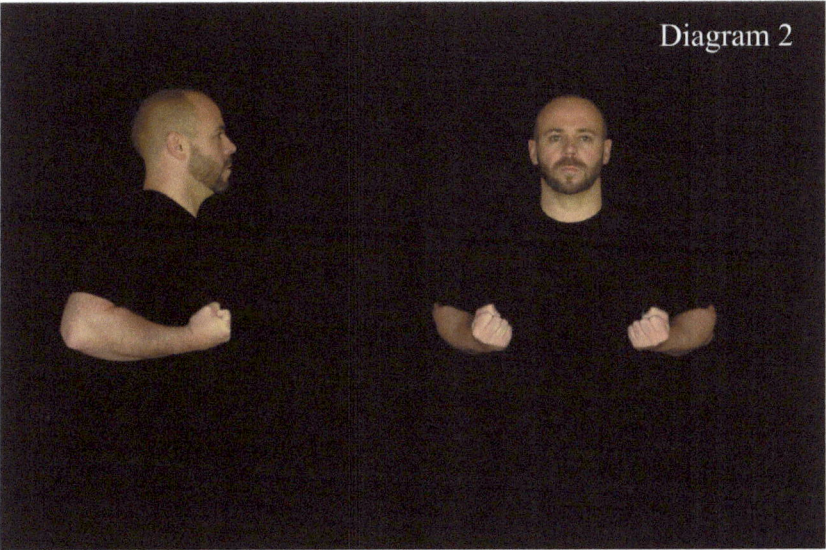

Diagram 2

Open the hands into the push position as shown in diagram 3 and exhale through the mouth.

Drain the lungs until your arms are fully extended forwards at shoulder height as shown in diagram 4. This completes the forward point of the Cross.

From that position take a deep breath of air in through the nostrils, returning to the closed-hand position as shown in diagram 2, and repeat the exercise as instructed at the beginner level.

Whilst completing the exercise maintain your posture, keeping your shoulders back, knees slightly bent, chin out, and eyes focused straight ahead.

A good tip for keeping good posture whilst initially performing this exercise is to face a full length mirror. This method will also provide you with assistance on focus; however, as soon as you are comfortable with your training position and posture do not rely any further on the mirror.

Continue the exercise as detailed in diagram 3 and 4 and please ensure that you adhere to the recommendations as shown below:

- Beginner: complete the exercise one to three times.
- Intermediate: complete the exercise five to ten times.
- Advanced: complete the exercise ten to twenty times.

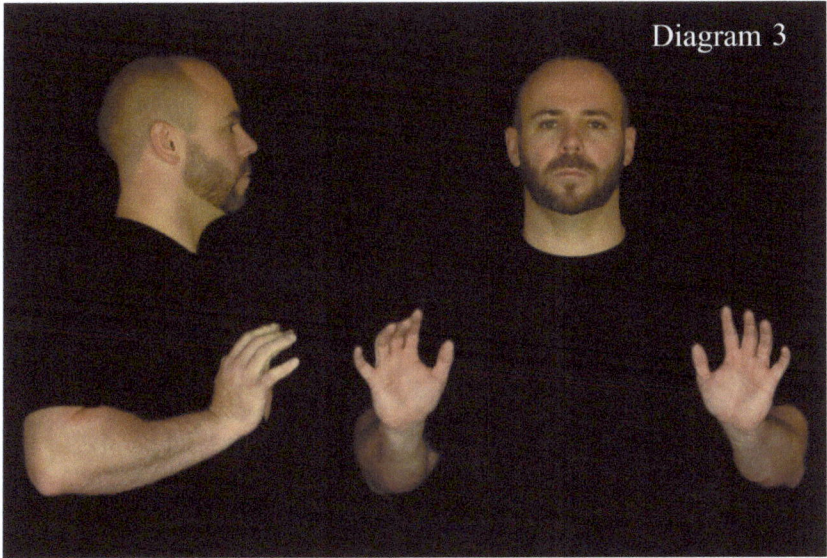

Diagram 3

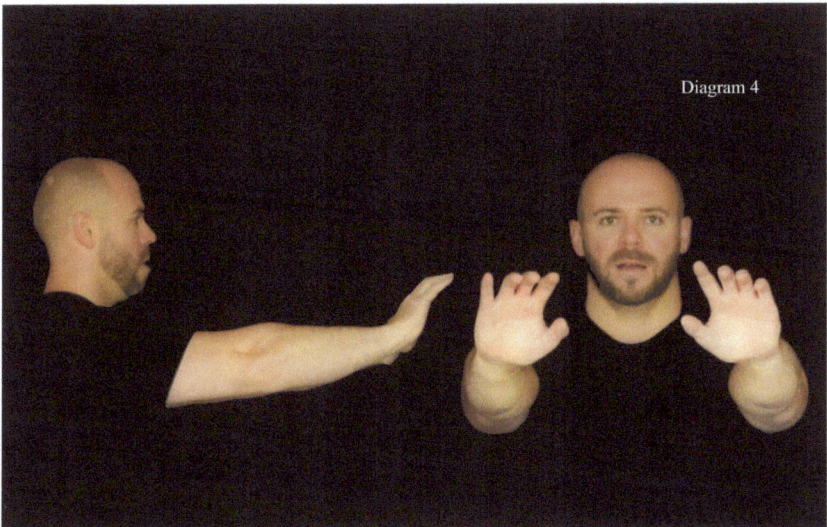

Diagram 4

Upward Point

Adopt the training posture with your hands open and arms fully outstretched at waist height as shown in diagram 5.

Pull your arms back to the closed-hand position at the side of the ribs, and whilst doing so take in a deep breath of air through the nostrils, filling the lungs and holding for approximately two seconds as shown in diagram 6.

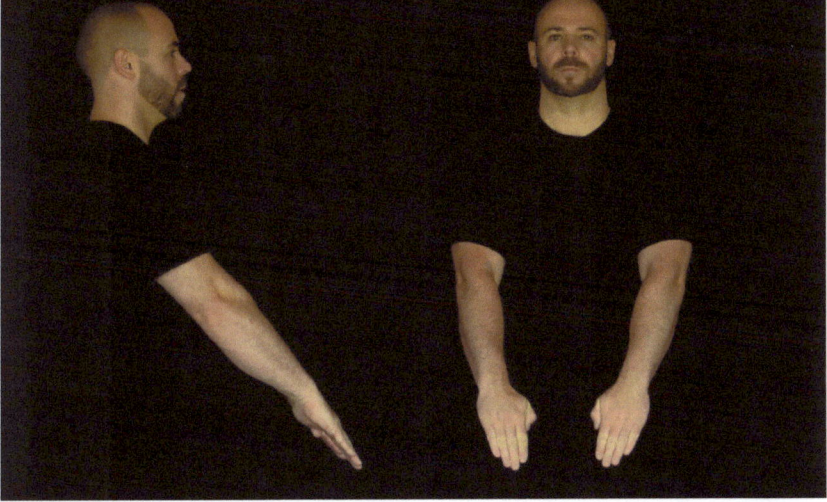

Diagram 5

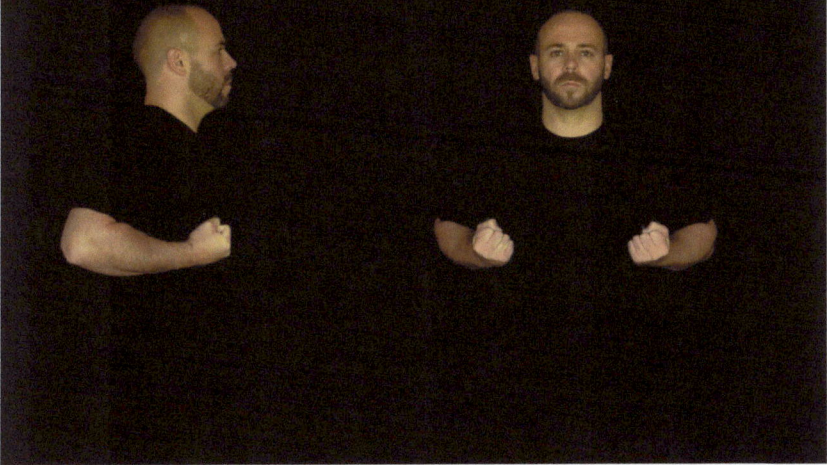

Diagram 6

Open the hands into the push position prior to looking upwards as shown in diagram 7.

Now look upwards, leaning the head backwards. Open your mouth wide and exhale, draining the air from the lungs slowly until your arms are fully extended upwards. Keep your hands in the push position, as shown in diagram 8, in order to complete the exercise.

From that position take a deep breath of air in through the nostrils, whilst returning to the closed-hand position as shown in diagram 6, and repeat the exercise as instructed at the beginner level.

Continue the exercise as detailed in diagrams 7 and 8 and please adhere to the recommendations as shown below:

- Beginner: Complete the exercise one to three times. If however you are feeling dizzy or disorientated please rest, and perhaps do this particular exercise in a seated position until you feel more confident. If the dizziness or disorientation continues in the seated position it is advised that you seek medical advice.
- Intermediate: complete the exercise five to ten times.
- Advanced: complete the exercise ten to twenty times.

In order to acquire the well-being of My-Chi, it is possible to achieve all or most of the exercises in a seated position, if a person is unable to stand for whatever reason.

We must strive to be the best we can be with whatever we have within ourselves.

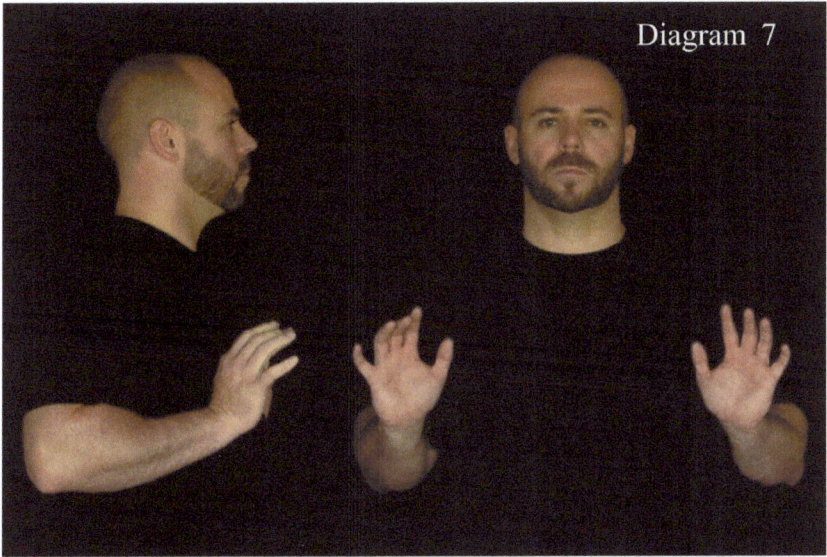

Diagram 7

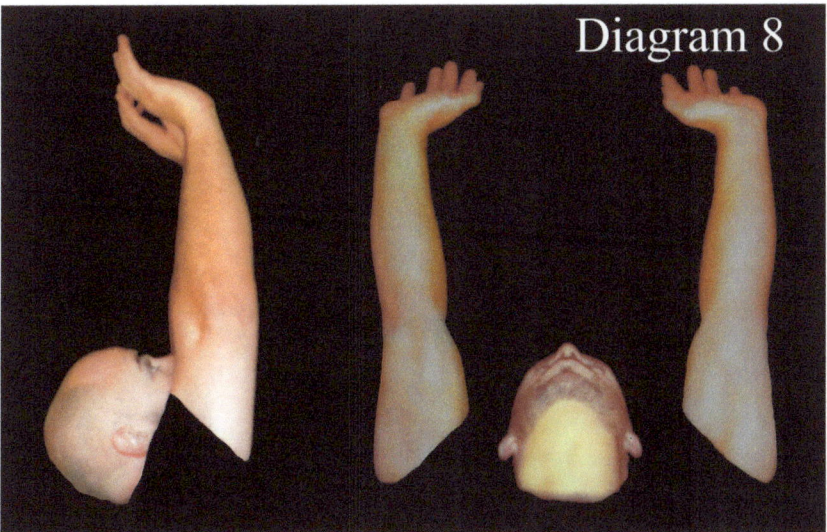

Diagram 8

THE POWER OF MY-CHI

Sideward Point

Once again adopt the training posture. Keep your eyes focused straight ahead, your hands open and arms fully outstretched at waist height as shown in diagram 9.

Pull your arms back to the closed-hand position at the side of the ribs. Whilst doing so take in a deep breath of air through the nostrils, filling the lungs and holding for approximately two seconds, as shown in diagram 10.

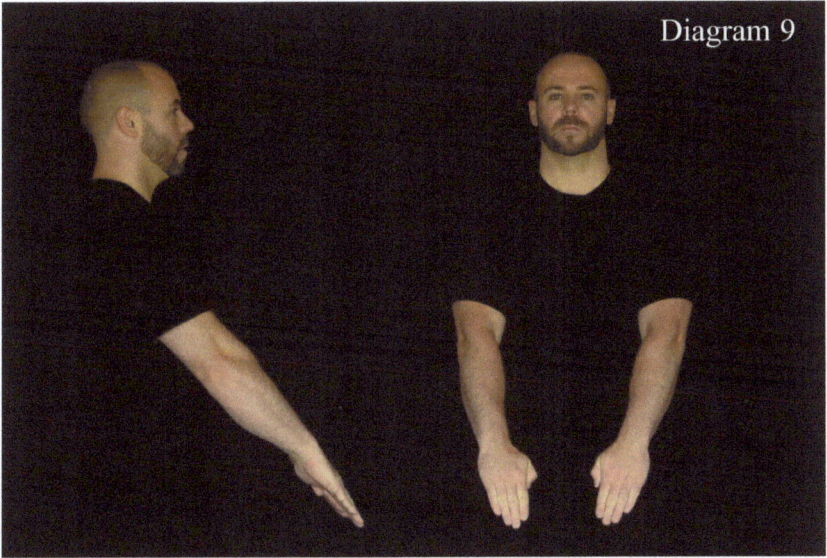

Diagram 9

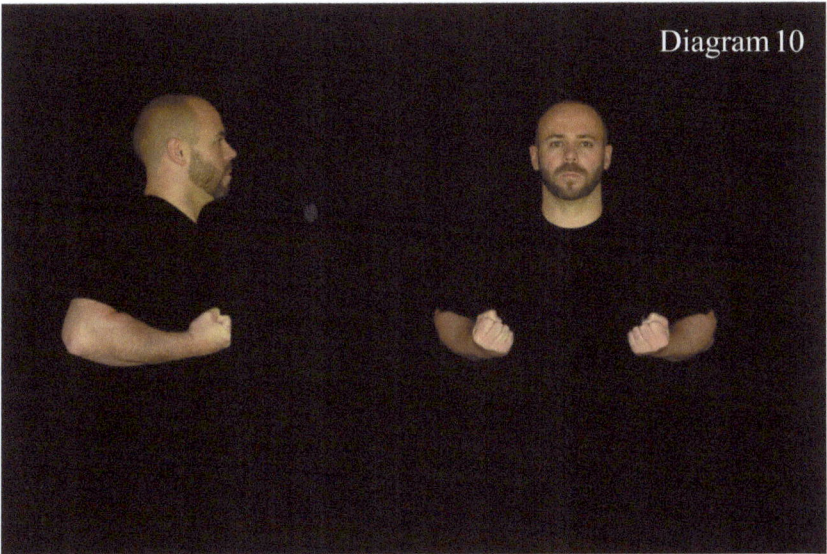

Diagram 10

Open the hands into the push position (diagram 11) while looking straight ahead.

Exhale through the mouth, draining the air from your lungs slowly until your arms are fully extended to the side, pushing the chest slightly forward, arms at shoulder height as shown in diagram 12.

From that position take a deep breath of air in through the nostrils whilst returning to the closed-hand position as shown in diagram 10. Repeat the exercise as instructed at beginner level.

Continue the exercise as detailed in diagrams 11 and 12 and please adhere to the recommendations as shown below:

- Beginner: complete the exercise one to three times.
- Intermediate: complete the exercise five to ten times.
- Advanced: complete the exercise ten to twenty times.

The sideward point will assist in the development of posture.

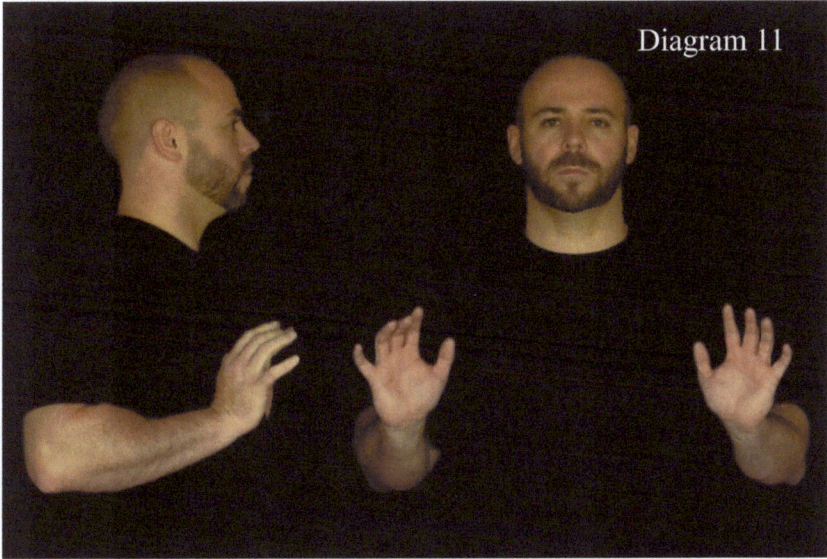

Diagram 11

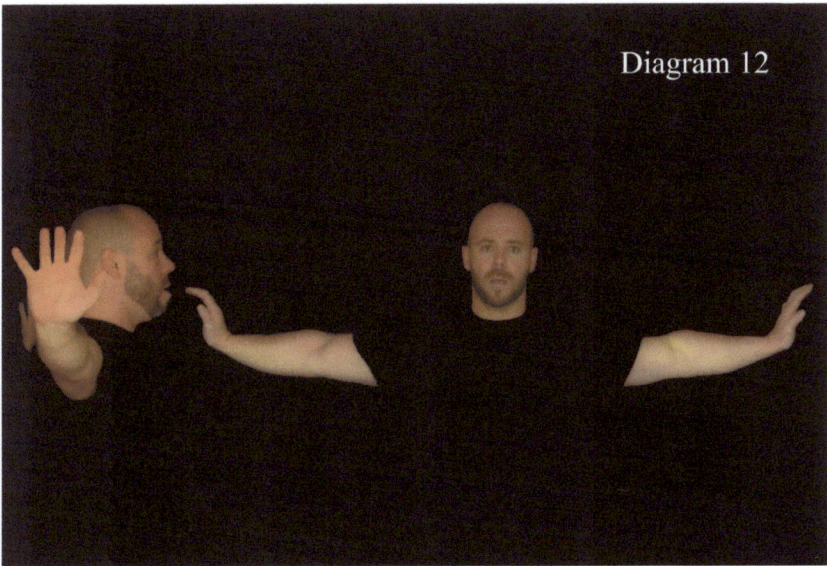

Diagram 12

DESCENDING POINT

Once again adopt the training posture. Keep your eyes focused straight ahead, your hands open, and your arms fully stretched at waist height as shown in diagram 13.

Pull your arms back to the closed-hand position at the side of the ribs. Whilst doing so take a deep breath of air, in through the nostrils and into the lungs, and hold for approximately two seconds as shown in diagram 14.

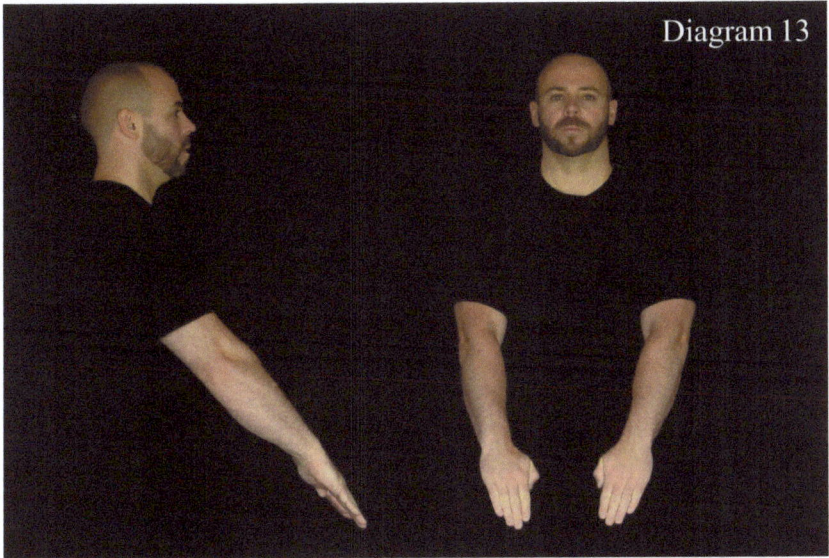

Diagram 13

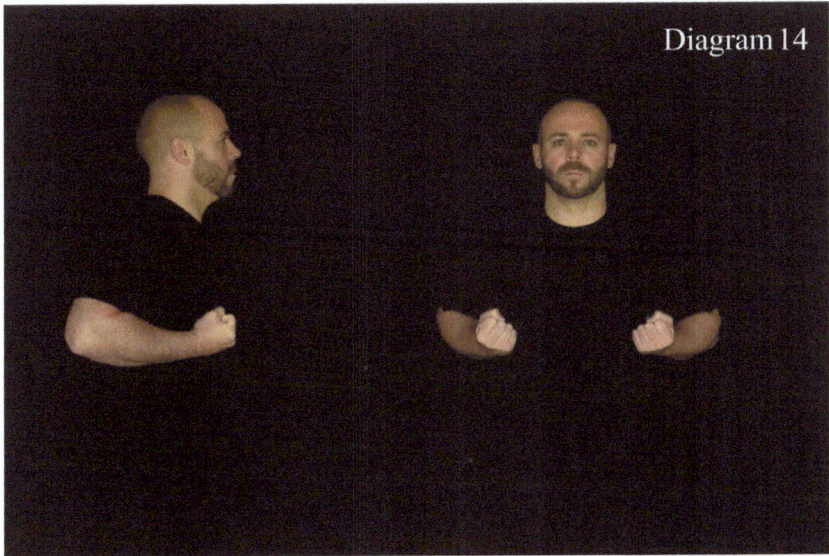

Diagram 14

Open the hands into the push position as shown in diagram 15, looking straight ahead throughout the descending point.

Exhale through the mouth, draining the air from your lungs slowly, until your arms are fully extended beyond the waistline as shown in diagram 16, in order to complete the exercise.

From that position take a deep breath of air in through the nostrils, returning to the closed-hand position as shown in diagram 14. Repeat the exercise as instructed at the beginner level.

Continue the exercise as detailed in diagrams 15 and 16 and please adhere to the recommendations as shown below:

- Beginner: complete the exercise one to three times.
- Intermediate: complete the exercise five to ten times.
- Advanced: complete the exercise ten to twenty times.

You may find yourself slowly and gradually looking downwards whilst doing this particular exercise. Practice well on your focus and you will eventually master it.

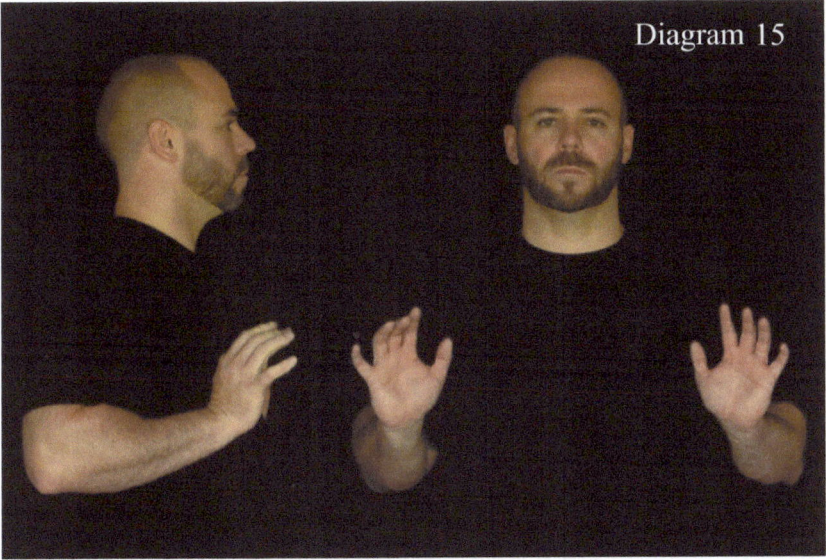

Diagram 15

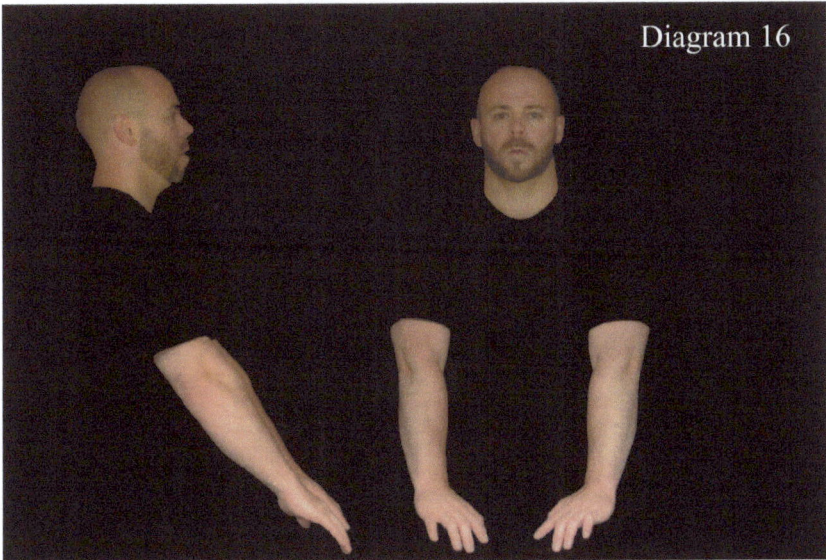

Diagram 16

You have now gone through all of the movements of the Cross. Continue to master this exercise before moving on to the Wall.

Life has made many of us slaves to the speed of modern day living, yet here is a golden opportunity to develop your well-being, through your own endeavours and at your own pace.

Practice well and you will begin to understand the power of the self; you will feel the confidence of My-Chi, and others will notice the newfound inner strength that is now a part of who you are.

The Wall

The second set of techniques come under the category of the Wall. It is essential that you have practiced the Cross well and understand the power of My-Chi before attempting the Wall. To train hard and often is good, but without the foundation of the basic techniques you may as well attempt to gather the wind.

The exercise of the Wall will take approximately three minutes to complete; however, as you are now a practiced student you may wish to slow down your technique in order to acquire the correct feeling, using the negative and positive muscles. To understand the negative and positive muscles, visualise a board with a strong coiled spring behind it. The positive muscle will push forward whilst the negative muscle will hold back the movement, giving you a sense of actually pushing against a powerful, resistant object.

With your hands in the open position you must push forward while breathing out, using the positive and negative muscle in order to have total control of the movement. Your hands will be at your target point (approximately 6-8 inches from the body) as you finish your exhalation, therefore it is essential that you push from the diaphragm and release a quicker, shorter breath than you did during the Cross exercise.

As your hands reach the target point, imagine that you are actually pushing against an immovable wall, and hold that position until you have exhaled and emptied the lungs.

Controlled breathing and body movement combined with inner Chi will oxygenate the whole body, including the muscles. Whilst training the Wall you must also maintain your basic training of the Cross, as you will lose the essence of My-Chi and an imbalance will occur, rendering your exercises useless and possibly harmful.

Forward Point

Standing in your training posture with your hands open and your arms fully stretched out at waist height as shown in diagram 17, pull your arms back with the hands in the closed position at the side of the ribs.

Whilst doing so take in a deep breath of air, through the nostrils into the lungs, and hold for approximately two seconds as shown in diagram 18.

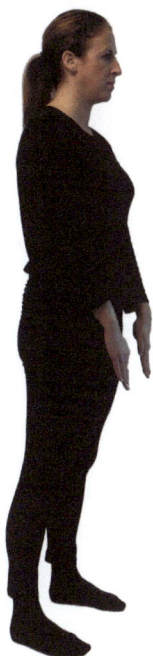
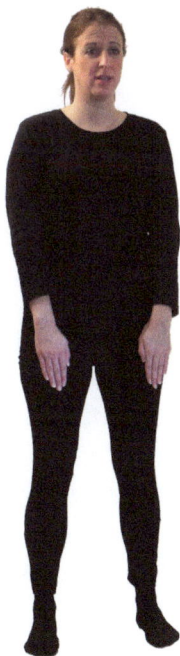

Diagram 17

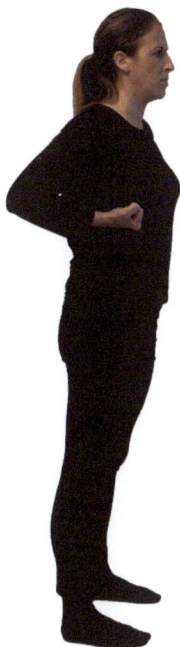
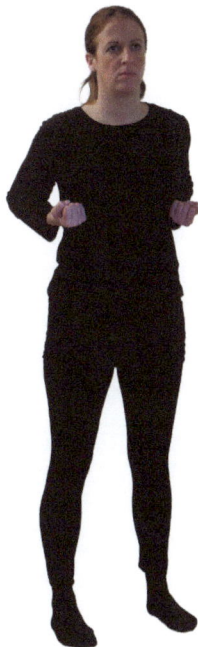

Diagram 18

Open the hands into the push position as shown in diagram 19. Focus your eyes straight ahead throughout the forward point, and exhale through the mouth.

Drain your lungs, using the diaphragm to force the air out quickly as the hands move forward at chest height, stopping against the Wall approximately 6-8 inches from your chest, as shown in diagram 20.

From that position take a deep breath of air in through the nostrils, returning to the closed-hand position as shown in diagram 18, and repeat the exercise as instructed at the beginner level.

Continue the exercise as detailed in diagram 19 and 20 and please adhere to the recommendations as shown below:

- Beginner: complete the exercise one to three times.
- Intermediate: complete the exercise five to ten times.
- Advanced: complete the exercise ten to twenty times.

Now that you have attempted the Wall you may realize that it is much more difficult than it appears.

Stand in your training posture, open your hands at the side of your ribs, take a deep breath of air in through the nostrils, and hold for approximately two seconds. Now exhale through the mouth using the diaphragm to assist in pushing the air out quickly from the lungs as the hands move forward at chest height, stopping against the wall approximately 6-8 inches from your chest. Now bring your closed hands back to the ribs, open the hands, and repeat the exercise until you have mastered the technique.

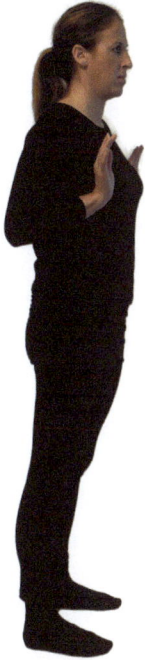
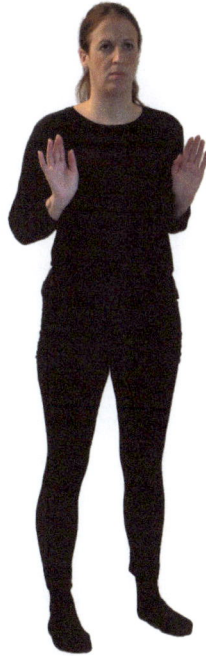

Diagram 19

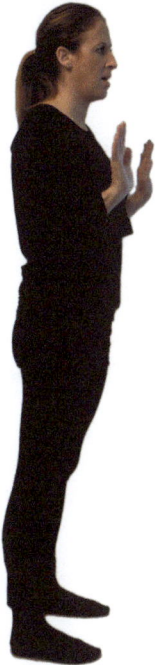
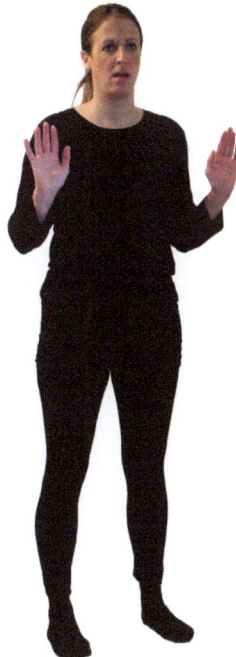

Diagram 20

It is very important that you take the time to understand the feeling of the Wall, so please practice the forward point well before moving on. I highly recommend that you rest after three repetitions, and begin again when you feel confident enough to do so. It is important that you imagine the Wall in front of you, approximately 6-8 inches from your body, and that you feel the resistance of that wall as you push against it at the end of your technique.

Ensure that you have mastered the whole of the technique from the start position as shown in diagram 17, to the finish position as shown in diagram 20, before moving on to the descending point.

Descending Point

Standing in your training posture with your hands open and arms fully stretched at waist height as in diagram 21.

Pull your arms back with hands in the closed position up to the side of the ribs and whilst doing so take in a deep, long breath of air, through the nostrils, into the lungs, and hold for approximately two seconds as shown in diagram 22.

The Power of My-Chi

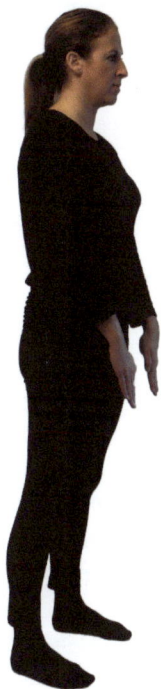
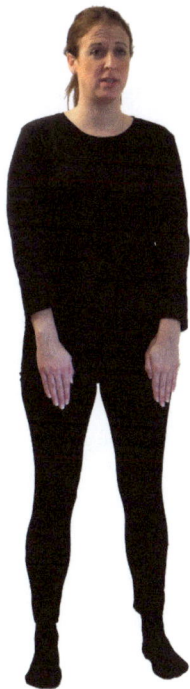

Diagram 21

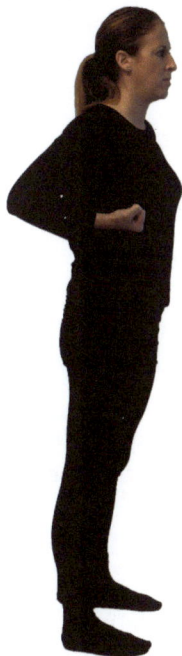
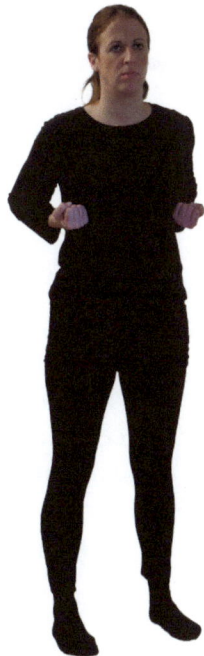

Diagram 22

Open the hands into the push position as shown in diagram 23.

With your eyes focused straight ahead, rotate the hands (fingers pointing upwards) and then quickly drop them to the side of your hips. Exhale through the mouth as you push the hands slowly forward, level with the hips and up against the Wall, approximately 6-8 inches from your body as shown in diagram 24.

From that position, take in a deep breath of air through the nostrils, returning to the closed-hand position as shown in diagram 22, and repeat the exercise as instructed at the beginner level.

Continue the exercise as detailed in diagram 23 and 24 and please adhere to the recommendations below:

- Beginner: complete the exercise one to three times.
- Intermediate: complete the exercise five to ten times.
- Advanced: complete the exercise ten to twenty times.

Whilst pushing the air out of the lungs during training the descending point, you must tighten the upper legs and buttocks. Once mastered this will assist when you move on with your training and progress to the Orb. Be sure to practice this well.

Once you have practiced the above and maintained the training posture and harmony of mind, body, and spirit, you will then be ready to move on to the sideward point.

Please note in the sideward point, as in diagram 26, that when the closed hand returns to the side of the ribs, the thumbs are tight against the ribs and the hands move out to the side in the ready position.

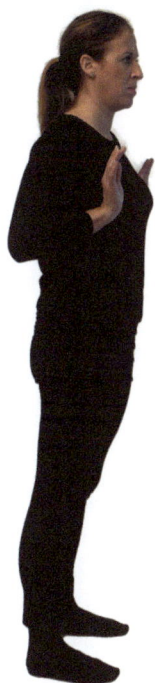
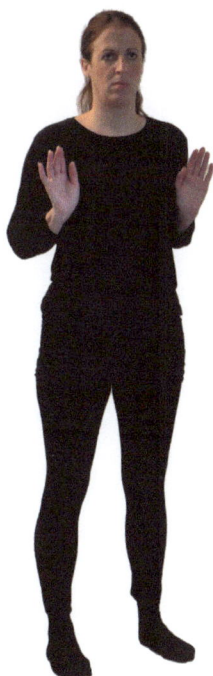

Diagram 23

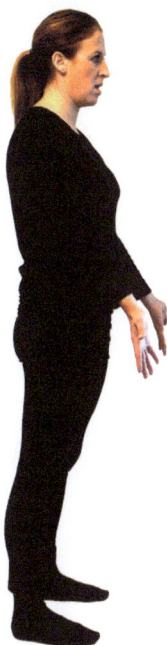
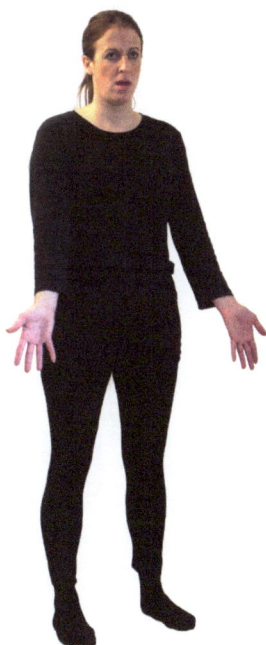

Diagram 24

SIDEWARD POINT

Standing in your training posture with your hands open and arms fully stretched at waist height as shown in diagram 25, pull your arms back with hands in the closed position, ensuring that on this occasion the thumbs are tight against the ribs.

Whilst doing so take in a deep breath of air through the nostrils, into the lungs, and hold for approximately two seconds as shown in diagram 26.

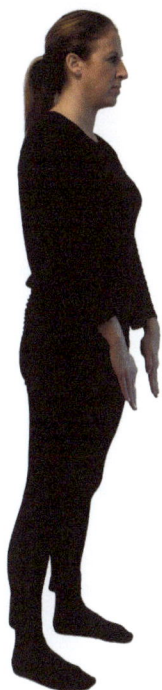 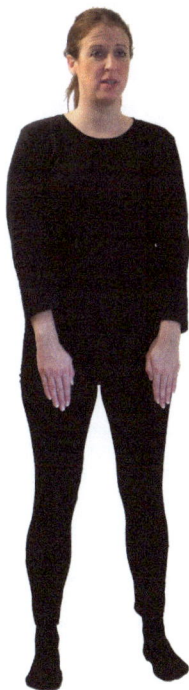

Diagram 25

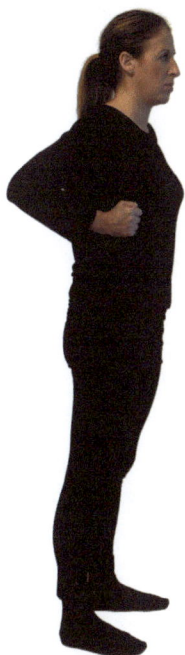 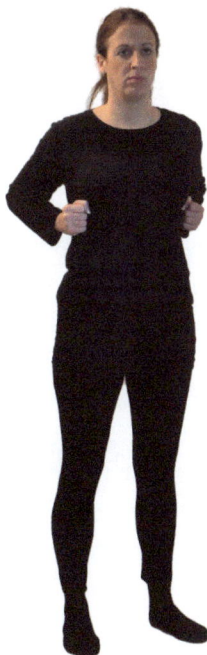

Diagram 26

Open the hands into the push position as in diagram 27 and quickly rotate the hands to the side, fingers pointing outwards.

Exhale through the mouth as you push the hands slowly forward, level with the stomach/diaphragm, and up against the Wall approximately 6-8 inches forward of your body as shown in diagram 28.

Remember to use the diaphragm in order to force the air out quickly on the sideward point exercises.

From this position take a deep breath of air in through the nostrils, returning to the closed-hand position as shown in diagram 26, and repeat the exercise as instructed at the beginner level.

Continue the exercises as detailed in diagrams 27 and 28 and please adhere to the recommendations as shown below:

- Beginner: complete the exercise one to three times.
- Intermediate: complete the exercise five to ten times.
- Advanced: complete the exercise ten to twenty times.

Whilst exercising the Wall sideward point try to pull the elbows back as far as possible, opening up the rib cage and filling the lungs with air to maximum capacity.

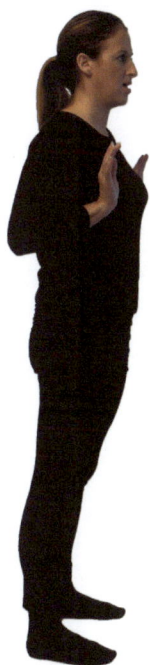
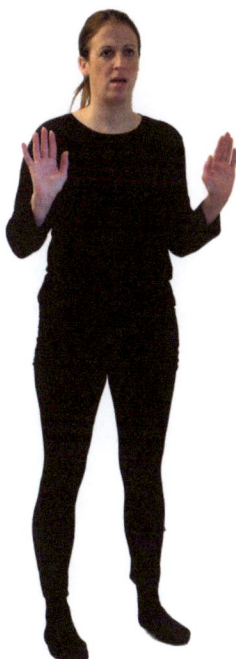

Diagram 27

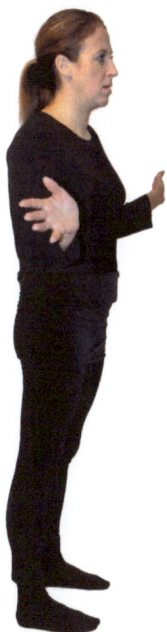
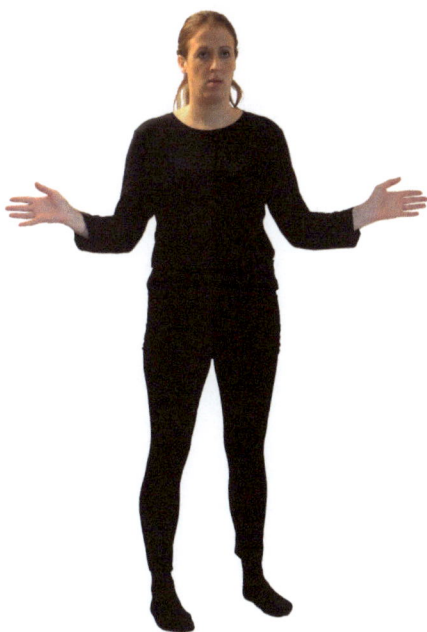

Diagram 28

Upward Point

Stand in your training posture with your hands open and arms fully outstretched at waist height as shown in diagram 29. Pull your arms back, with hands in the closed position, up to the side of the ribs.

Whilst dong so take in a deep, long, controlled breath of air in through the nostrils, into the lungs, and hold for approximately two seconds, as shown in diagram 30.

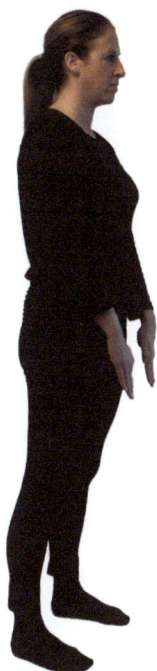 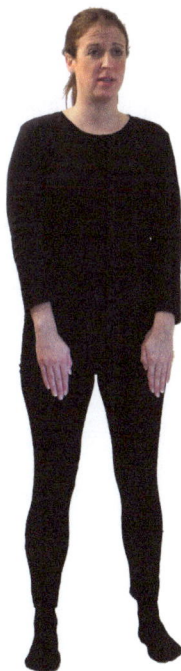

Diagram 29

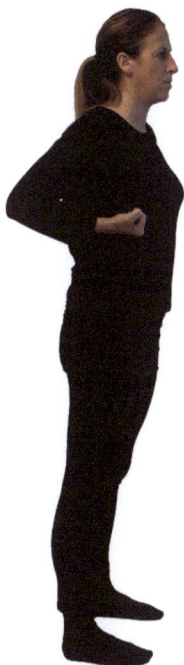 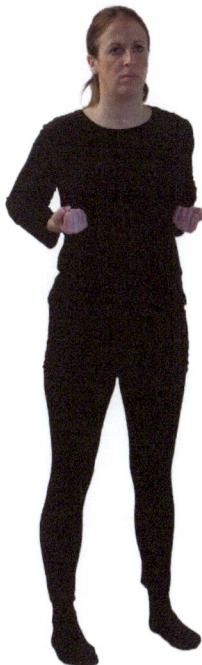

Diagram 30

Open the hands into the push position as shown in diagram 3.

Looking straight ahead, raise the hands quickly to head height, then exhale as you push the hands slowly forward, level with your head and up against the Wall approximately 6-8 inches from your body as shown in diagram 32.

Continue the exercise as detailed in diagrams 31 and 32 and please adhere to the recommendations as shown below:

- Beginner: complete the exercise one to three times.
- Intermediate: complete the exercise five to ten times.
- Advanced: complete the exercise ten to twenty times.

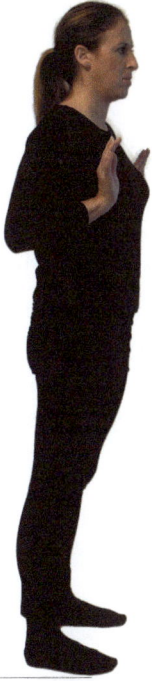
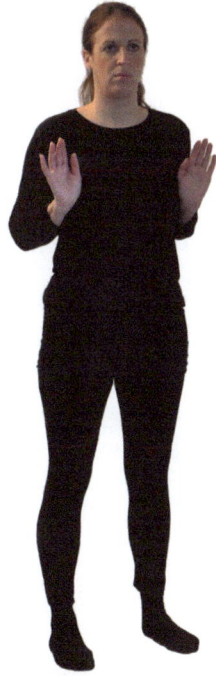

Diagram 31

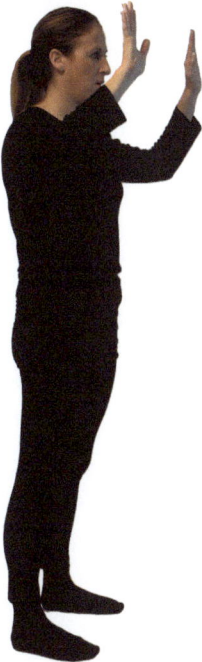
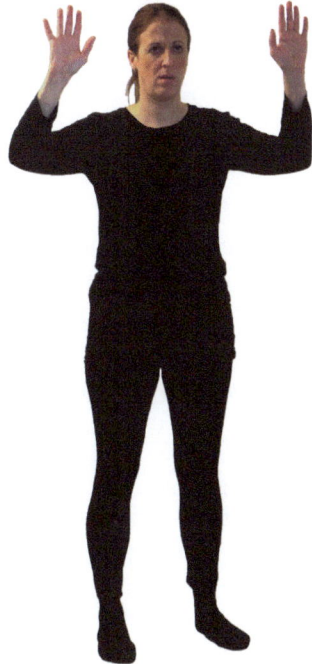

Diagram 32

Reversed Descending Point

For the following exercise you must imagine that the Wall is now approximately 6-8 inches to your rear. You will swing the arms forward from the open hand position quickly to alongside your upper leg, after which you will exhale the air from your lungs whilst pushing slowly approximately 6-8 inches to the rear of the body as shown in diagram 36.

Ensure that whilst exhaling you tighten the upper thighs and buttocks as you push the air out assisted by the diaphragm. This development is essential as you progress further on to the exercise of the Orb.

Standing in your training posture with your hands open and arms fully outstretched at waist height as shown in diagram 33, pull your arms back with hands in the closed position at the side of the ribs. Whilst doing so take in a deep breath of air through the nostrils, into the lungs, and hold for approximately two seconds as shown in diagram 34.

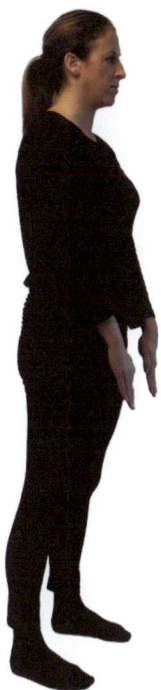
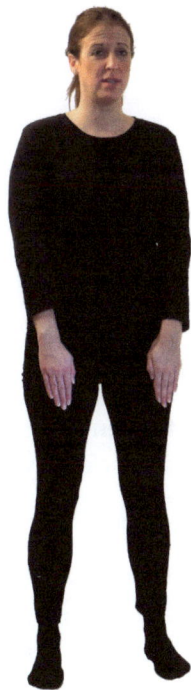

Diagram 33

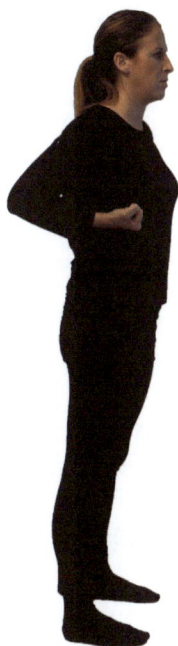
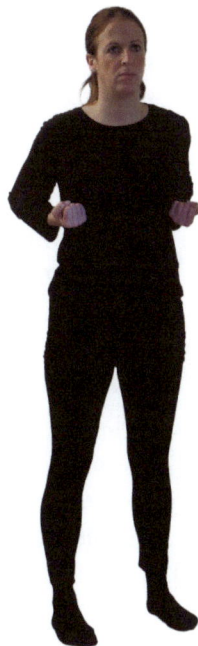

Diagram 34

Open the hands into the push position as shown in diagram 35. Focus the eyes straight ahead throughout the Reversed Descending Point, swinging the arms gently forward until they are straight and level with the side of the upper leg.

Exhale through the mouth, draining the air quickly from the lungs with the diaphragm, tensing the upper legs and buttocks as you push the hands approximately 6-8 inches to the rear of the body as shown in diagram 36.

From that position take a deep breath of air in through the nostrils, returning to the closed-hand position as shown in diagram 34 and repeat the exercise as instructed at the beginner level.

Continue the exercise as detailed in diagrams 35 and 36 and please adhere to the recommendations as shown below:

- Beginner: complete the exercise three to five times.
- Intermediate: complete the exercise five to ten times.
- Advanced: complete the exercise ten to fifteen times.

Once again I must remind you to practice regularly the Cross and the Wall in order to maintain and achieve the best of My-Chi.

Please now take the time to exercise My-Chi and enjoy the journey so far. There is no rush; you have a newfound energy and power available at your fingertips. It has always been with you, it just needed to be harnessed by way of My-Chi.

The third set of techniques, if you are ready, come under the category of the Orb.

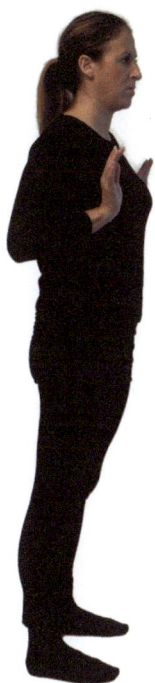
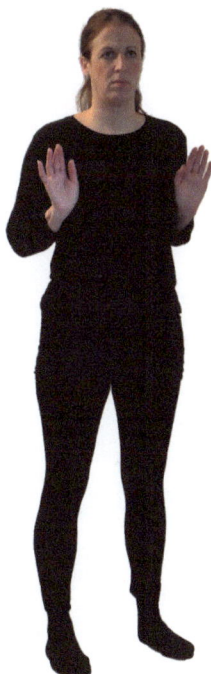

Diagram 35

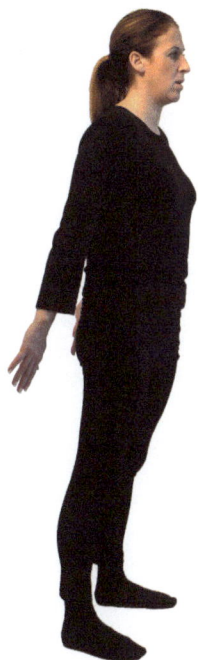
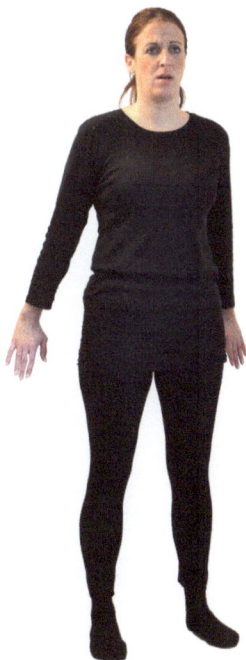

Diagram 36

You have now gone through all of the movements of the Wall. Continue to master this exercise before moving on to the Orb.

THE ORB

The Orb is for advanced students. The concentration of these exercises is aimed at the inner organs such as liver, kidneys, etc. The posture, as well as the arm and hand movements, of the following techniques focuses on those inner organs; however, at this advanced stage of your training you will simultaneously and automatically, through your breathing technique, stimulate the whole of the body with My-Chi. Once you have mastered the Orb, you will have the ability to concentrate My-Chi upon those organs by way of inner massage and stimulation, dispersing oxygenated blood to those areas.

I must reiterate once again that in order to practice and understand the Orb, you must be fully trained and familiar with the Cross and the Wall. All of these exercises are laid out in progressive order and must be followed as prescribed.

The Orb exercise consists of a movement similar to that of the Wall, insomuch as you are visualizing an Orb that is situated about a foot in front of you. Imagine that it is roughly the size of a football and that its centre is just below the sternum.

Remember the Orb is not the energy, your Chi is the energy. The Orb is merely an imaginary object upon which you can concentrate your Chi. You will now start to feel the energy of Chi passing from your hands and into the Orb from each angle that you perform the exercise.

You must remember to maintain your training position, concentrating the mind, body, and spirit with your Chi breathing, and be sure to force the air out when exhaling with the diaphragm.

The Two-handed Orb

Top Point

Standing in your training posture with your hands open and arms fully outstretched at waist height as shown in diagram 37, pull your arms back with hands in the closed position at the side of the ribs.

Whilst doing so take in a deep long breath of air through the nostrils, into the lungs, and hold for approximately two seconds as shown in diagram 38.

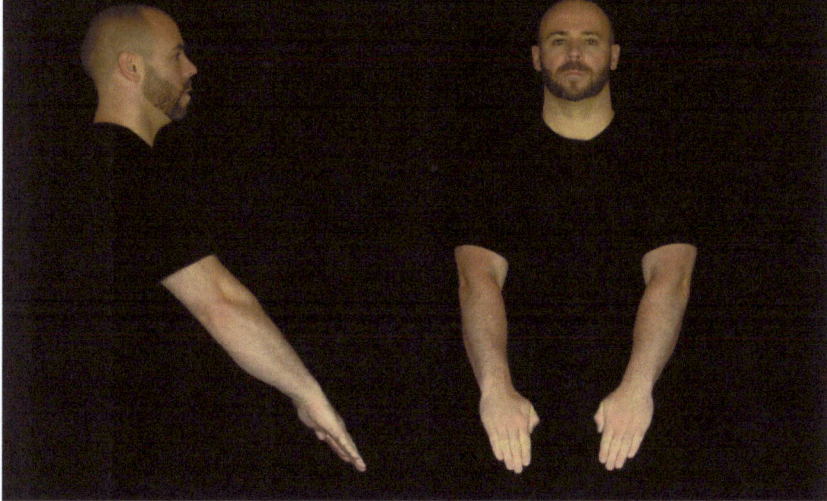

Diagram 37

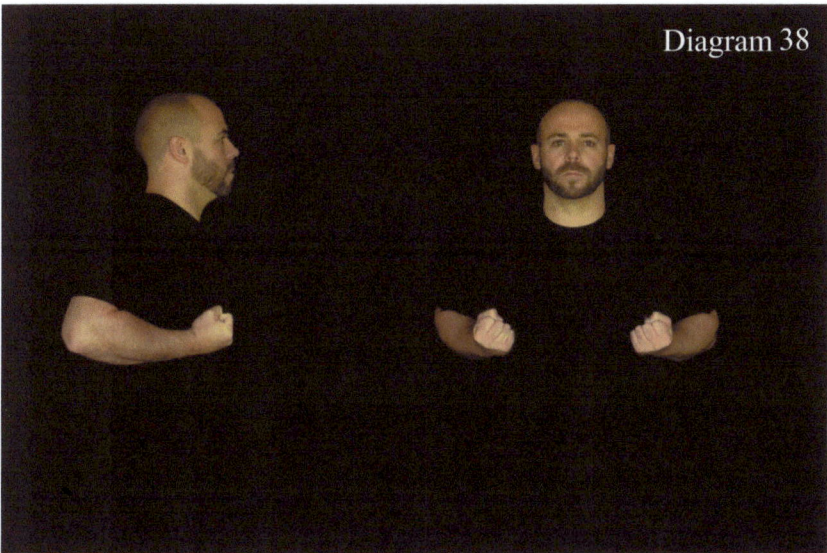

Diagram 38

Open the hands into the push position as shown in diagram 39.

Focus your eyes straight ahead throughout the Top Point, exhale through the mouth, draining the air from your lungs slowly until your hands meet the top of the Orb, as shown in diagram 40.

From that point take in a deep breath of air through the nostrils, returning to the closed-hand position as shown in diagram 38, and repeat the exercise as instructed at the Orb beginner level.

Continue the exercise as detailed in diagrams 39 and 40 and please adhere to the recommendations as shown below:

- Beginner: complete the exercise two to three times.
- Intermediate: complete the exercise three to four times.
- Advanced: complete the exercise four to five times.

Remember that you are now concentrating your Chi into the Orb; however, you also ought to be feeling the energy in the stomach area whilst doing this exercise as by now you are well-trained in the art of breathing My-Chi, which at this level is automatically sending freshly oxygenated blood to every component of your body.

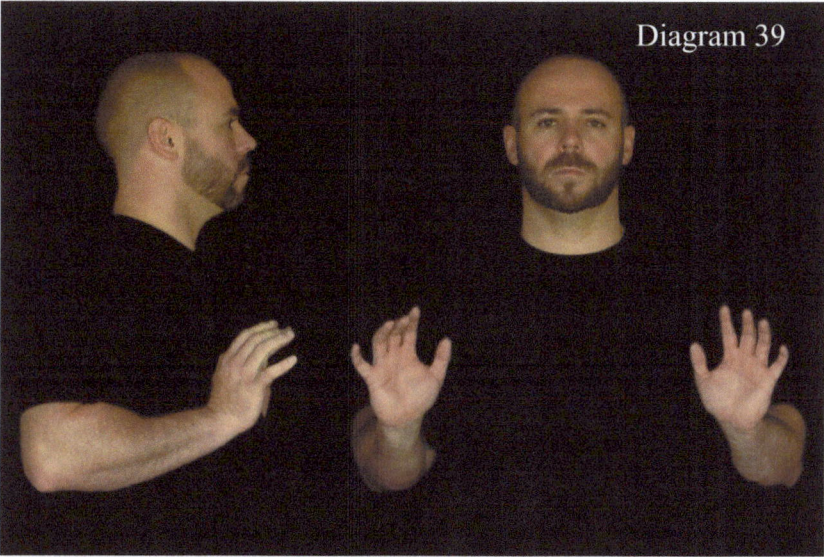

Diagram 39

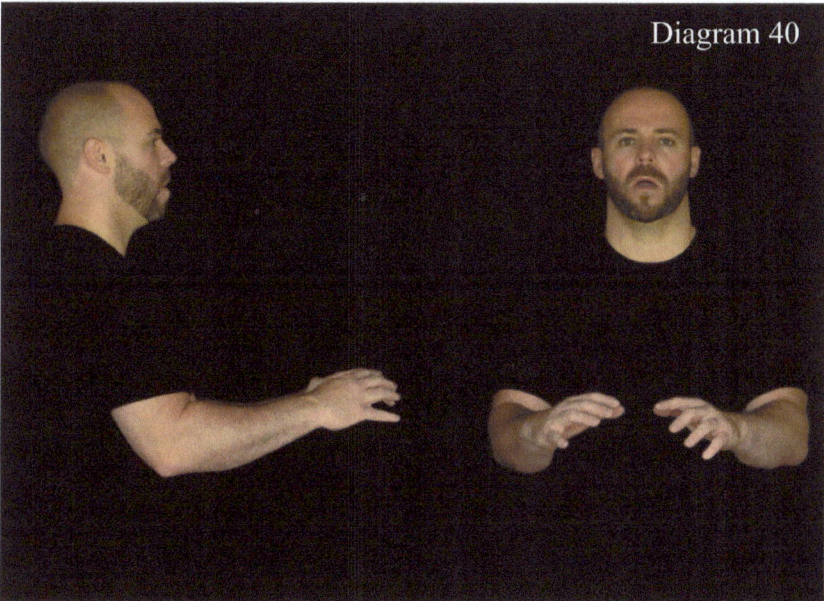

Diagram 40

SIDEWARD POINT

Standing in your training posture with your hands open and arms fully outstretched at waist height as shown in diagram 41, pull your arms back with hands in the closed position at the side of the ribs.

Whilst doing so take in a deep breath of air through the nostrils, into the lungs, and hold for approximately two seconds as shown in diagram 42.

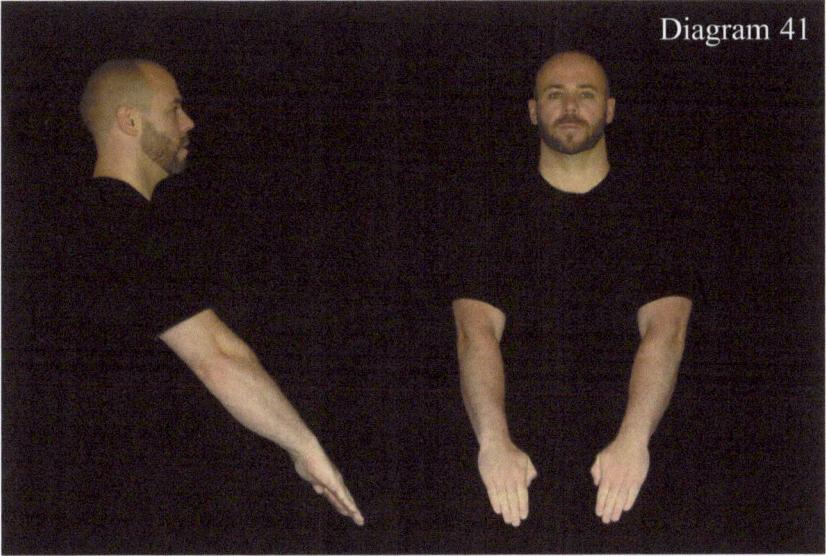

Diagram 41

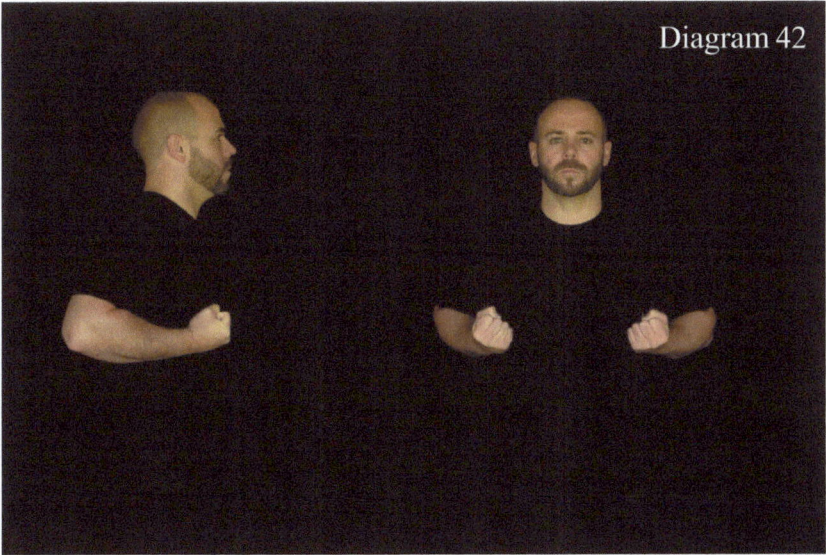

Diagram 42

Open the hands into the push position as shown in diagram 43.

Keep your eyes focused straight ahead throughout the Sideward Point, exhale through the mouth, draining the air slowly from your lungs assisted by the diaphragm, until your hands meet the side of the Orb, as shown in diagram 44.

From that position take a deep breath of air in through the nostrils whilst returning to the closed-hand position as shown in diagram 42, and repeat the exercise as instructed at the beginner level.

Continue the exercise as detailed in diagrams 43 and 44 and please adhere to the recommendations as show below:

- Beginner: complete the exercise two to three times.
- Intermediate: complete the exercise three to four times.
- Advanced: complete the exercise four to five times.

The Orb ought to be familiar to you now; however, if you feel that you have not quite got the feel of it, then practice those two techniques again before moving on to the final two-handed technique of the Orb Lower Point.

Remember the position of the Orb that you are visualising about a foot from your body and anticipate well the lower position before attempting the exercise.

You may once again find yourself looking down occasionally whilst doing this exercise; practice it until you are confident enough to do this exercise while maintaining your training posture.

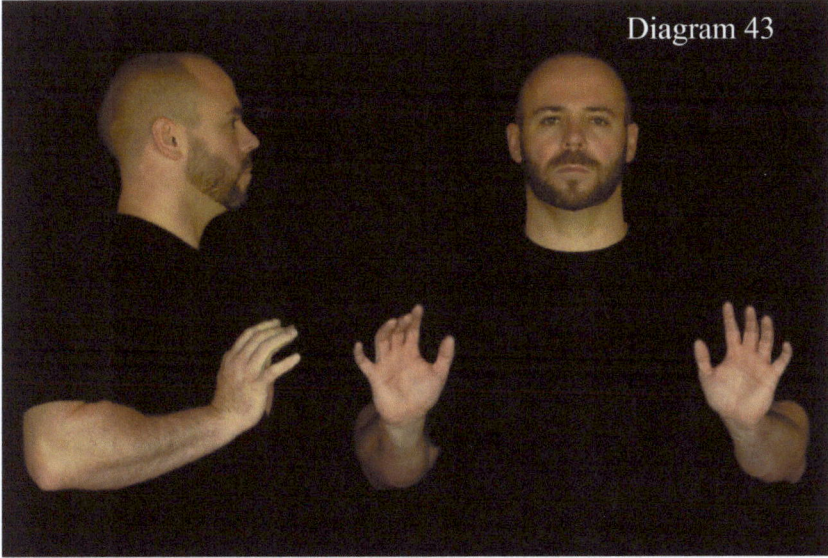

Diagram 43

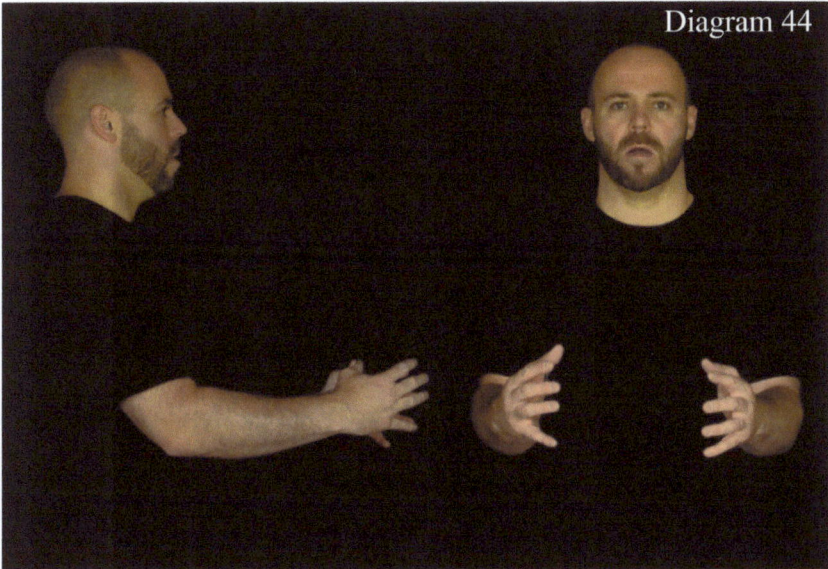

Diagram 44

LOWER POINT

Standing in your training posture with your hands open and arms fully outstretched at waist height as shown in diagram 45, pull your arms back with hands in the closed position at the side of the ribs.

Whilst doing so take in a deep, long breath of air through the nostrils, into the lungs, and hold for approximately two seconds as shown in diagram 46.

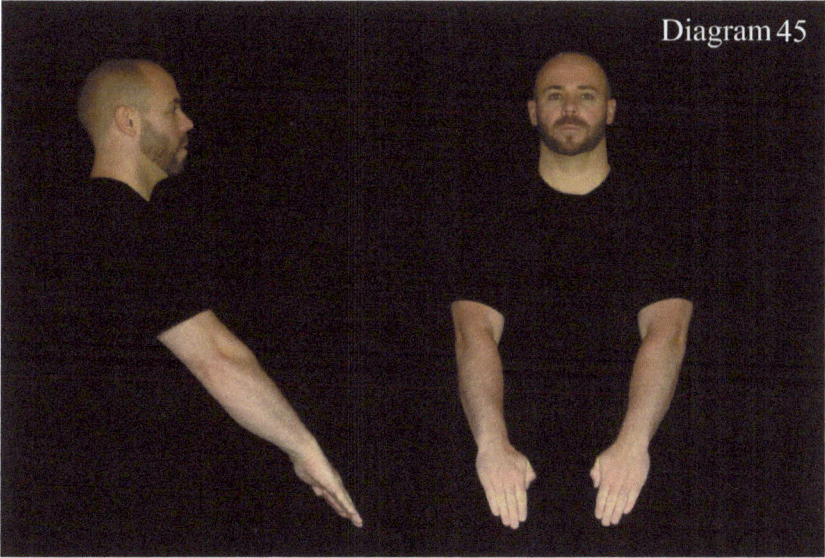

Diagram 45

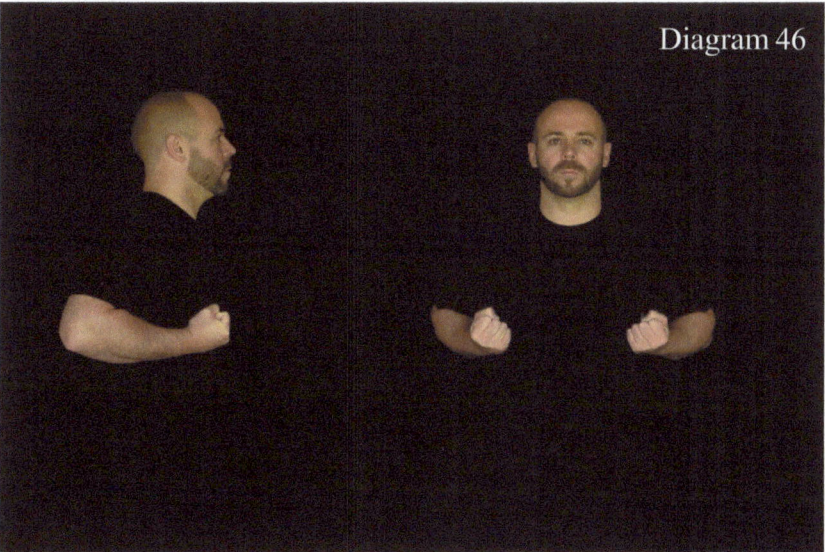

Diagram 46

Open the hands into the push position as shown in diagram 47. Keep your eyes focused straight ahead throughout the Lower Point, exhale through the mouth, draining the air from the lungs slowly, whilst rotating the hands outward and bringing them under the Orb.

At this point you will have then emptied the air from your lungs to complete the exercise as shown in diagram 48.

From that position take a deep breath of air through the nostrils whilst returning to the closed-hand position as shown in diagram 46, and repeat the exercise as instructed at the beginner level.

Continue the exercise as detailed in diagrams 47 and 48 and please adhere to the recommendations as shown below:

- Beginner: complete the exercise three to four times.
- Intermediate: complete the exercise four to five times.
- Advanced: complete the exercise five to six times.

Now is a good time to practice all three exercises of the Two-handed Orb. Take your time to master this technique before moving on to the One-handed Orb.

You must practice the one-handed movement of the Orb casually at first in order to understand the movement – left hand out and return, and then right hand out and return – thus switching the Chi from one hand to the other.

When you have mastered this movement only then is it time for you to move on and continue with the final phase of instruction in this book.

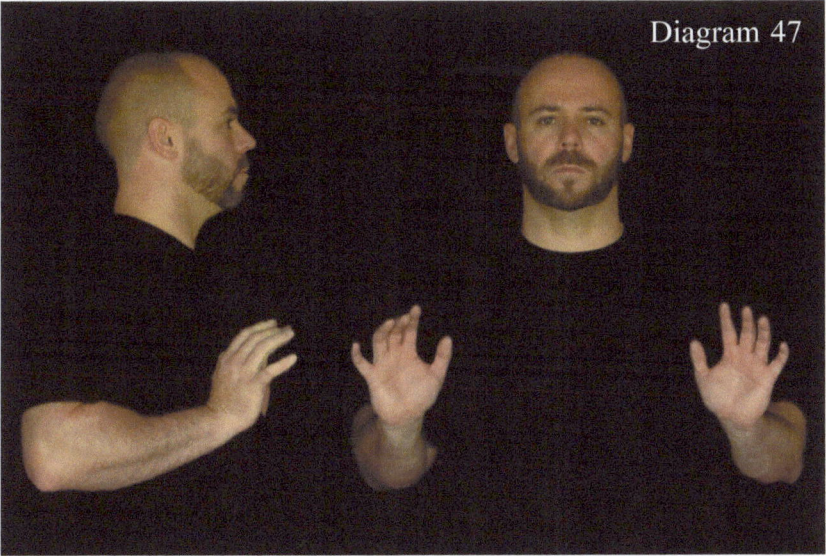

Diagram 47

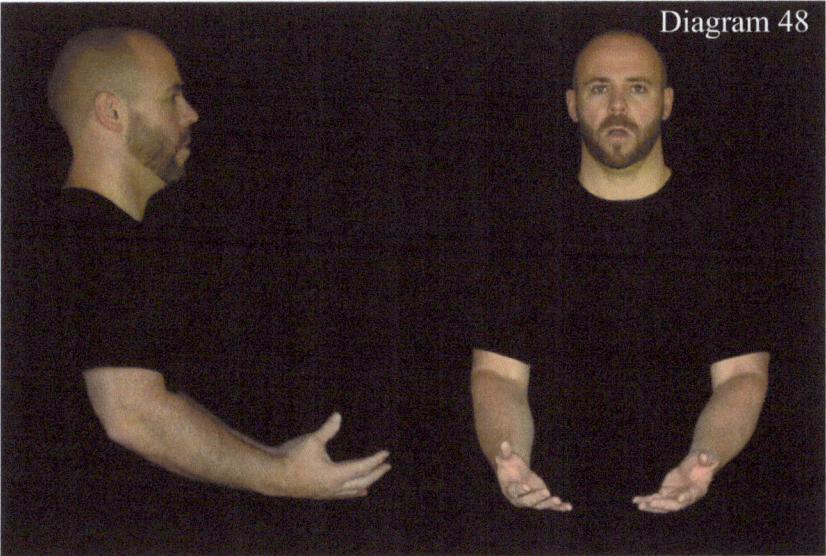

Diagram 48

The One-handed Orb

Standing in your training posture with your hands open and arms fully outstretched at waist height as shown in diagram 49, pull your arms back with the hands in the closed position at the side of the ribs.

Whilst doing so take in a deep, long breath of air through the nostrils, into the lungs, and hold for approximately two seconds, as shown in diagram 50.

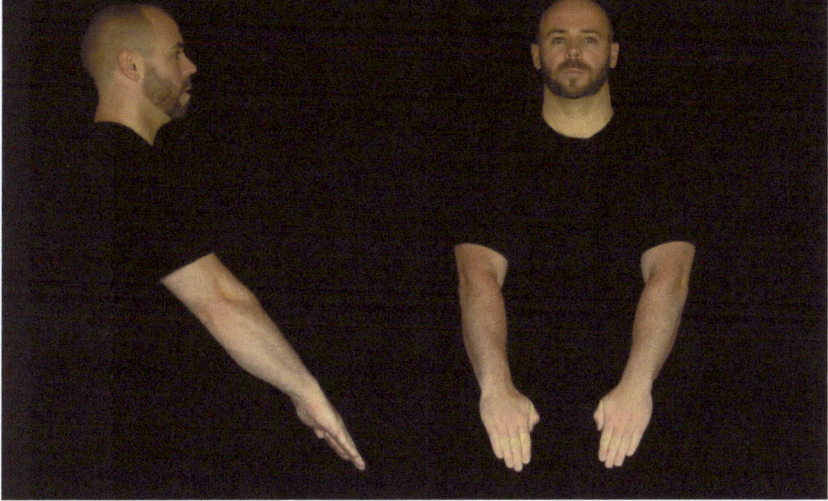

Diagram 49

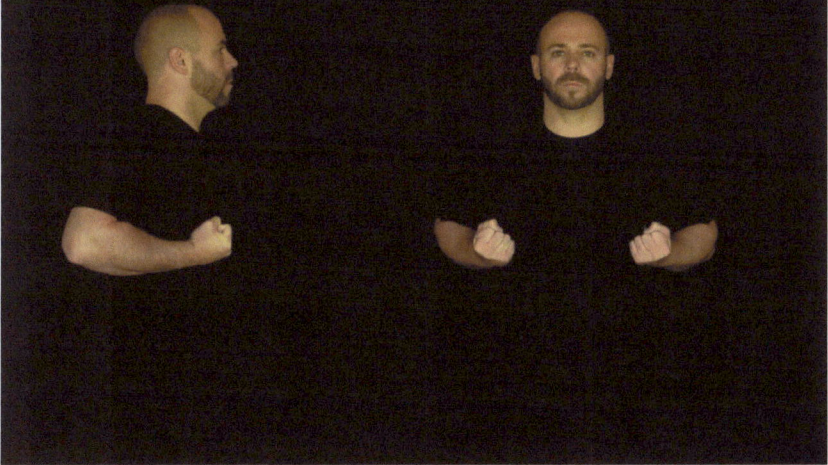

Diagram 50

Open the left hand into the push position as shown in diagram 51.

Keep your eyes focused straight ahead throughout the one-handed point, exhale through the mouth, draining the air slowly from the lungs as you reach out in front of the body, level with the stomach until your arm is fully extended and pressing against the single imaginary Orb, as shown in diagram 52.

From that position take a deep breath of air in through the nostrils whilst returning to the closed-hand position as shown in diagram 53.

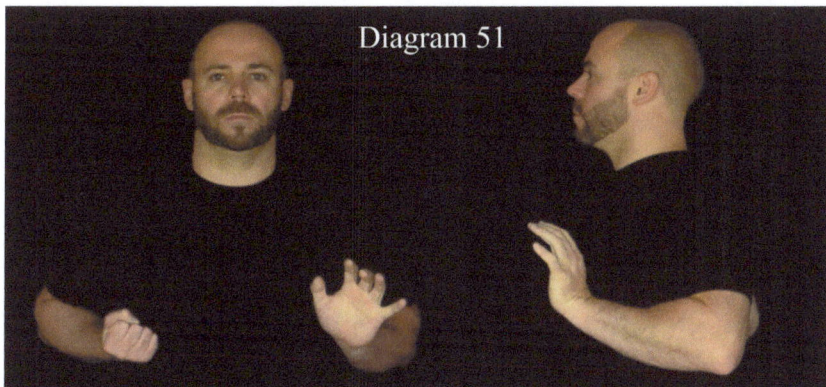

Diagram 51

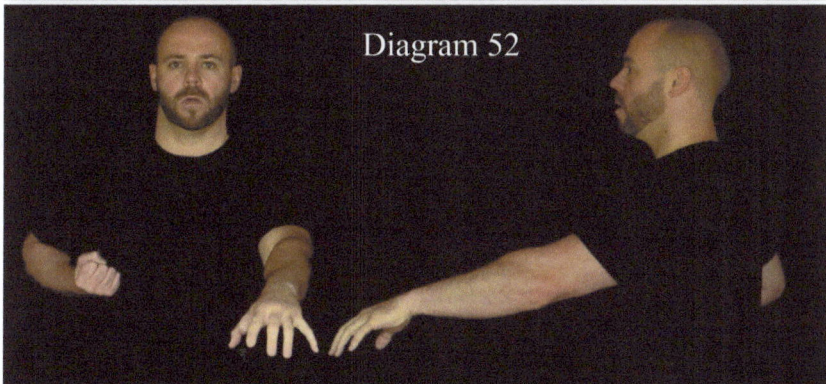

Diagram 52

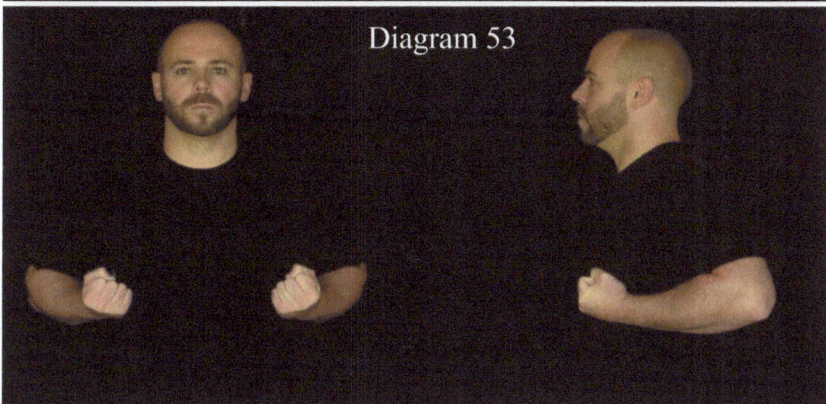

Diagram 53

Now change to the right hand as shown in diagrams 54 to 56. Repeat the exercise, alternating from right to left and left to right and so on as instructed at the beginner level.

Continue the exercise as detailed in diagrams 51, 52, and 53, and please adhere to the recommendations below:

- Beginner: complete the exercise four to six times.
- Intermediate: complete the exercise six to eight times.
- Advanced: complete the exercise eight to ten times.

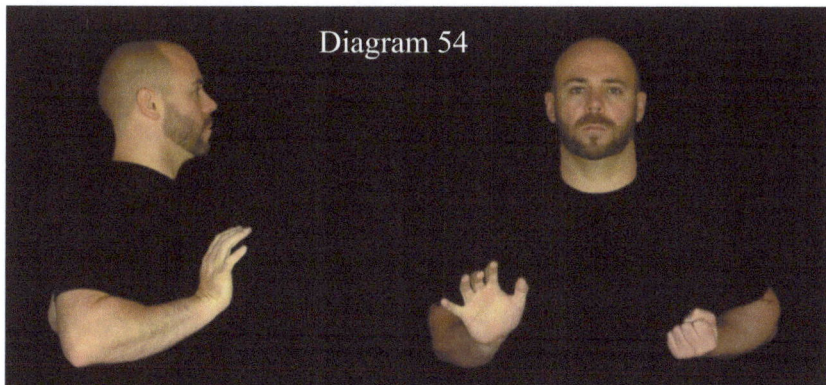

Diagram 54

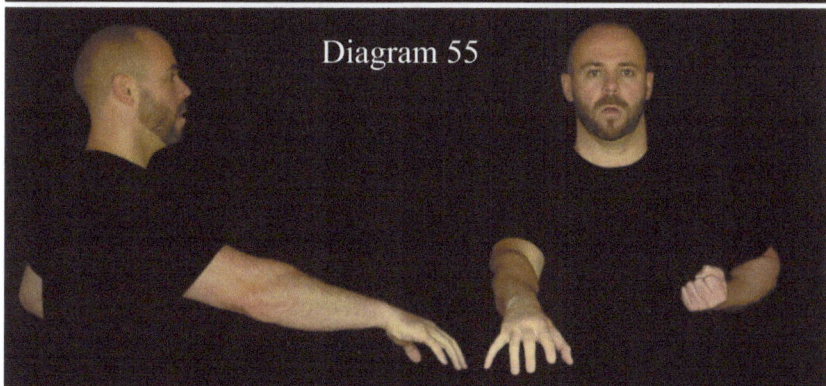

Diagram 55

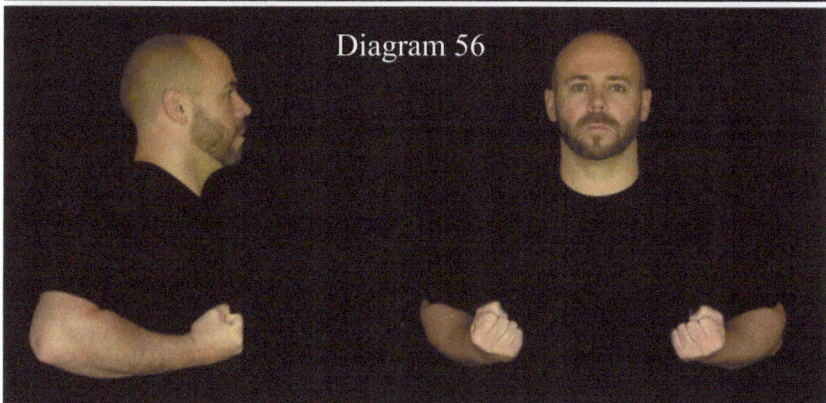

Diagram 56

W elcome to the world of My-Chi! You have exercised from the Cross to the Orb and if you have practiced well, you will now know the true feeling of My-Chi/Your-Chi.

The one-handed Orb is proof that you can channel your Chi into whatever part of the body you choose.

Check out your posture, body toning, inner strength, feel-good factor – check out your total feeling of well-being.

If you have followed the instructions to the full then you, and your family and friends, will have noticed a phenomenal change in your overall being.

Continue to practice and develop My-Chi. You have found the gift that lies within you. It is yours.

There is no death, only a change of worlds.
[attributed to] Chief Si'ahl (Seattle)

LIFE'S MOUNTAIN

I have written briefly about my epic walks on the *Camino Santiago de Compostela* in Spain. My most difficult walk was the *Camino Sureste*, a nine hundred kilometre walk from San Pedro that took me past my villa in Campoverde on the Costa Blanca and ended in the town of Astorga in the province of Leon in northern Spain. It was during this Camino that I had the idea of writing "Life's Mountain"

After six days of walking the Sureste, I arrived at the sleepy village of Petrola. It had been a twenty-five kilometre hike that day; the sun was beating down and it was over eighty degrees and very humid. I called in at a local café bar and ordered myself a well-deserved beer. It was the perfect place to end my day, so I asked the owner if there was a place for pilgrims to rest for the night. He told me where I could get a key to the local church, a customary night's stopover for pilgrims to use along the way.

I managed to find the key holder who escorted me to the church and showed me where the pilgrims slept – a little room at the side of the main church in which there were two tables, a row of chairs, and some other artefacts obviously associated with church functions. I unpacked the clothes that I would wear the following day, had a shower, and set up my sleeping bag on one of the tables as I felt that the floor would be too hard and cold. Afterwards, I set off to find a place to eat. On the other side of the village I found the San Juan Restaurant where I had the *menu de del dia* (menu of the day), a three-course meal for as little as eight euros. The meal was plentiful and beautifully cooked. Whilst I was there, the proprietor of the restaurant told me that he had also walked the Camino Sureste and showed me the certificate that he had acquired, which was proof that yes indeed he, too, had been on this same pilgrimage.

After my meal I returned to my room at the church and sat for a while, contemplating the generosity of the people in this little village – people who had given me shelter for nothing, fed me for a little monetary return, and been friendly to this stranger in their village. It was truly humbling and I was feeling good about life.

I went through My-Chi exercises and then sat with my diary, trying to get a full and comprehensive detailed outline on life. I began to write "Life's Mountain" there in that little annex to the church, comparing life to my challenges on the Camino: the preparation required at the beginning, the anticipating of all eventualities, the planning of my route, and making sure I was well equipped for what possibly lay ahead.

Over the following weeks, in the evenings, out there on the Camino Sureste whilst my mind was clear of other worldly influences and distractions, I eventually finished writing "Life's Mountain". My own climb, of course, goes on.

Life's Mountain

Each and every one of us must climb life's mountain. We all start at the bottom: rich, poor, able-bodied or disabled – we all start at the beginning, at the foot of a colossal journey. This journey will prove who we are by way of how we approach the ascent and by which path we decide to take in order to reach the top.

Some will falter before the ascent through no fault of their own. The journey is just not meant to be. Those who remain will begin to climb of life's mountain. Of those, some will have guidance along the way from parents, friends, mentors, and many other types of helpers who will make the climb easier when it becomes difficult to progress.

Some will chose not to listen to these helpers. They will feel the need to find their own way, to make their own mistakes, to discover on their own the path they wish to take, be it right or wrong, difficult or easy. This could be a good, character-building method, one that teaches a person independence of thought, and how to live with the consequences of their choices.

On the other hand, there will be those who will need to learn how to approach each stage of the climb without the advantage of others sharing their experiences of life's mountain. However, as they reach higher levels of the climb, this disadvantage will become a strength. They will progress by way of their well-practiced judgement, dealing with issues and problems that arise along the way single-handedly. If they manage to reach the top of life's mountain, then they will have a sense of self-achievement that only they and those of a similar disposition will appreciate.

Some will look with awe and dread at the task ahead, and will approach life's mountain with great trepidation. They will have doubts as to their ability to progress: will they fall, can they succeed, will they keep up with the others who are setting out, are they capable of taking on such a task, what lies ahead, what could befall them along the way. With or without the advice of others, theirs will be the hardest mountain to climb, because they will not enjoy the experience of the journey. When and if they arrive at the top, they will look back and feel cheated by the opportunities that others had taken, opportunities they themselves had avoided and rejected, excitement and adventure they had failed to embrace as they climbed life's mountain.

Despite all of this, or even because of it, how can we enjoy the journey of experiences that is life's mountain to the fullest?

The Beginning

Life's Mountain can be a long, drawn out climb for many people, one that lasts decades or, for some, more than a century. Before we set out on our journey, it is important that we plan the route, that we look at the path we intend to take and analyse any possible pitfalls. Listen to others that are at different stages of the ascent, ask them what difficulties they experienced at certain stages of the climb, and what they would choose to do differently if they were about to begin from where you are now standing.

How do they perceive the next stage of their climb? Are they on the right path or have they faltered and lost their way, and if so why? Tell them of your intentions, listen to their criticisms and also to their advice, for they have been where you are now standing. Take from them and benefit from their experiences, listen to their words of wisdom as they relate their experiences both good and bad. This will help you to make good decisions along the way.

Speak to your contemporaries. Ask them how they perceive the journey, what are their ambitions, fears, expectations, do they also have a plan, will they have some form of assistance, do they feel as though they will need assistance, are they ambitious as to what they want to achieve along the way? Over a short period of time you will build up a picture of others' intentions regarding their climb. This will broaden your scope and outlook regarding your own journey, and of how you intend to climb your own life's mountain.

Whilst on your journey you might alter the original plan as you progress, modify it or because of some unforeseen circumstances adjust it slightly. However, you must try to stick with the main essence of your plan. Do not falter – minor adjustments may be necessary, but you must stay the course. If you prepare well, you will have time to enjoy the journey with confidence, as opposed to wasting time resolving problems that occur because of your lack of preparation.

THE ASCENT

When you are fully prepared to climb life's mountain and you have chosen the route you wish to take, you must maintain complete awareness as you take each step. Look at your surroundings and enjoy your journey. There is no great hurry to reach the top, as there are many at the top who would give up everything in order to start again at the beginning.

After so many steps, stop for a while and look at the perspective you have gained from a higher elevation. Assess your progress and be honest with yourself. Have you travelled along the correct path, or have you faltered and strayed a little? Now is the time to reflect, and to correct any mistakes you have made. Prepare for the next stage of your journey; remain focused, and do not be tempted by the many distractions which may lead you away from your objectives.

Observe those around you, compare your position to theirs – not in an egotistical, critical, or self-satisfied manner, but as a yardstick in order to determine if you are getting the most out of your journey to the top of life's mountain.

Try to find likeminded people to talk with, and perhaps join them on the next stage of your journey. You will meet many friends who will be of assistance to you along the way; enjoy their company, their opinions, their outlook, and their aspirations. Some will fall behind, but some will move on ahead. Choose carefully who you walk with as their influence could confuse your own objectives. Remain focused and follow your own way.

As you ascend life's mountain you will encounter many crossroads. Be sure that as you climb you are looking ahead and anticipating these crossroads well in advance of their approach. If you are prepared when reaching these crossroads, your decisions will be well-founded and you will move on with confidence.

Remember that whilst travelling you must take the time to stop and appreciate the journey along the way. Take time to reflect on the decisions you have made and the routes you have taken. Heed the fellow travellers to which you have spoken and listened, evaluate their opinions, consider their experiences and future ambitions, examine the route they have taken and how it compares to your own.

As you near the top of life's mountain you will see that some friends have not made the climb. Though they have fallen by the wayside, their memory can be enjoyed as you stop and reflect before moving on to the final ascent.

When you have finally reached the top of life's mountain, you may feel weary and spent. On the other hand, you may feel strong and positive. Either way, the most important and satisfying feeling is that you have made it to the top and have enjoyed the journey.

The Top

You have been fortunate enough to reach the top of life's mountain. It is time to sit and reflect, to remember each and every stage of the climb, the fellow travellers you have helped along the way, and those who have kindly helped you.

As you look back down life's mountain, you will see family and friends at their own particular level of the climb, searching for their own way, and as much as you may wish to give them a helping hand, you can only advise them as to how you would have, or possibly did approach their present situation at that stage of life's mountain. There will be those who will listen to your experienced views, and there will be those who will ignore the voice of experience. Now that you are at the top, you may find that those below cannot hear or understand you too clearly. They will inevitably make their own mistakes. However, there will be times when some do hear you and take your advice. You can then observe their progress with great satisfaction.

You may reflect on the good times and the bad times – you may even be amused by the times that were hard and appeared unbearable, the times that you perhaps felt you could no longer go on.

If you prepared well for your ascent up life's mountain, if you planned from the beginning and set goals to achieve, targets that you wished to reach, you can now see how those plans and targets may have changed along the way. Perhaps it may be that you did not falter along the way, that you remained focused and fortunate.

Looking back, from your elevated view on top of life's mountain, you will now see the crossroads and paths where you made the right decisions and of course those where you made the wrong decisions. You will have experienced many things along the way, and took on many challenges. Or, perhaps you avoided certain issues and certain tracks that you could have taken, had you been a little more adventurous.

Many of us at the top of life's mountain wish to start again at the beginning, carrying the knowledge and foresight that we have acquired through our experiences. I wonder would it have been as exciting if we'd known what was around every twist and turn of the path, if we'd had all of the answers, if we could have avoided the pains, thus watering down the pleasures, losing in the process that sense of adventure and wonderment, living instead in a world of predictability.

I doubt it very much.

The time will come when each and every one of us will leave life's mountain. We will see beyond the horizon that we have all of our lives been striving to reach.

We must leave behind those who continue to climb and those at the very top, but who knows – perhaps they will follow us on our next journey, as we may follow those who have gone before us. Maybe it has always been so.

When my time comes to leave life's mountain I will look forward to the next challenge, for although my mind and body will remain here on life's mountain, My-Chi – my energy, my life force, my spirit – will move on to whatever lies ahead.

ENERGY IS ETERNAL

BECOME A MY-CHI LIFESTYLE MEMBER

Some of the benefits of a My-Chi Lifestyle:

Improved posture
Develop inner strength
Become more motivated
Become more positive
Become more body-positive
Improve body toning
Stress relief
Controlled breathing
Improved health and well-being
Improved blood circulation
Lower blood pressure
Exercising the inner organs
Clarity of mind
Spiritual awareness
Self-awareness
Self-control
Positive mental attitude
Harnessed spirit and power
Eliminate aggression
Environmental awareness
Improved character and self-discipline
Improved self-confidence

Enjoy the benefits of communicating with us on our website. We are there to welcome you, offering you the full benefits of a My-Chi membership, which include:

Audible Instruction from Tom Sullivan.
Animated exacting movements.
One-on-one with Tom Sullivan.
Occasional philosophies.
Regular updates from Tom Sullivan's diary.
One-on-one with other students, networking.
Private instruction, discount for members.
Discount on all merchandise.
Advanced My-Chi exercises.
News about seminars/weekend training.
Talk to your local Mentors, ask for advice.
Find out how to become a Mentor.

Find us at www.my-chi.co.uk

www.ingramcontent.com/pod-product-compliance
Lightning Source LLC
Chambersburg PA
CBHW040929030426
42334CB00002B/15